Current Cardiovascular Therapy

Series editor
Juan Carlos Kaski
London, UK

Cardiovascular pharmacotherapy is a fast-moving and complex discipline within cardiology in general. New studies, trials and indications are appearing on a regular basis. This series created with the support of the International Society of Cardiovascular Pharmacotherapy (ISCP) is designed to establish the baseline level of knowledge that a cardiovascular professional needs to know on a day-to-day basis. The information within is designed to allow readers to learn quickly and with certainty the mode of action, the possible adverse effects, and the management of patients prescribed these drugs. The emphasis is on current practice, but with an eye to the near-future direction of treatment. This series of titles will be presented as highly practical information, written in a quick-access, no-nonsense format. The emphasis will be on a just-the-facts clinical approach, heavy on tabular material, light on dense prose. The books in the series will provide both an in-depth view of the science and pharmacology behind these drugs and a practical guide to their usage, which is quite unique. Each volume is designed to be between 120 and 250 pages containing practical illustrations and designed to improve understand and practical usage of cardiovascular drugs in specific clinical areas. The books will be priced to attract individuals and presented in a softback format. It will be expected to produce new editions quickly in response to the rapid speed of development of new CV pharmacologic agents.

Brendan Madden
Editor

Treatment of Pulmonary Hypertension

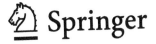 Springer

Editor
Brendan Madden
St George's Hospital
London
UK

ISBN 978-3-319-13580-9   ISBN 978-3-319-13581-6   (eBook)
DOI 10.1007/978-3-319-13581-6

Library of Congress Control Number: 2015947616

Springer Cham Heidelberg New York Dordrecht London

Printed on acid-free paper

Springer International Publishing AG Switzerland is part of Springer Science+Business Media (www.springer.com)

Contents

Contributors

Editor

Brendan Madden Division of Cardiac and Vascular Science, St. George's Hospital, London, UK

Contributors

Jenny Bacon Cardiothoracic Unit, St. George's Hospital, London, UK

Adam Loveridge Cardiothoracic Unit, St. George's Hospital, London, UK

Caroline Patterson Department of Respiratory Medicine, St. George's Hospital, London, UK

Laura Price Section of Vascular Biology, National Heart and Lung Institute, Imperial College, London, UK

Dongmin Shao Section of Vascular Biology, National Heart and Lung Institute, Imperial College, London, UK

Stephen John Wort Department of Pulmonary Hypertension, Royal Brompton Hospital, London, UK

Chapter 1
The Pathophysiology, Presentation and Diagnostic Investigation of Pulmonary Hypertension

Jenny Bacon and Brendan Madden

Introduction

The definition of pulmonary hypertension (PH) is an elevated resting mean pulmonary artery pressure (mPAP) of greater than or equal to 25 mmHg, determined by right heart catheterisation [1]. It is a progressive and ultimately fatal disease without appropriate management. Many different diseases can be associated with this elevation in mPAP and therefore PH is a diverse clinical entity.

J. Bacon
Cardiothoracic Unit, St. George's Hospital, London, UK
e-mail: jb901@doctors.org.uk

B. Madden (✉)
Division of Cardiac and Vascular Science,
St George's Hospital, London, UK
e-mail: brendan.madden@stgeorges.nhs.uk

B. Madden (ed.), *Treatment of Pulmonary Hypertension*,
Current Cardiovascular Therapy,
DOI 10.1007/978-3-319-13581-6_1,
© Springer International Publishing Switzerland 2015

1

PH can be broadly categorised into those conditions that are associated with the histological features of plexogenic pulmonary arteriopathy (PPA [2]) and those which are not. Conditions associated with PPA are grouped under the umbrella term pulmonary arterial hypertension (PAH). In PAH the left atrial pressure is usually normal, and is measured as the pulmonary wedge pressure (PWP) during right heart catheterisation (PWP <15 mmHg). The difference between mPAP and PWP is then divided by cardiac output to calculate pulmonary vascular resistance (PVR), and this is significantly elevated in PAH. Examples of diseases in the group PAH include idiopathic, heritable and PAH in association with certain drugs or toxins, scleroderma, human immunodeficiency virus (HIV) infection or portal hypertension.

Many patients develop PH in association with cardiopulmonary diseases. PH is commonly associated with left heart disease (such as mitral valve disease), chronic lung diseases (such as sleep disordered breathing, lung parenchymal and airway diseases) and chronic pulmonary thromboemboli (termed chronic thromboembolic pulmonary hypertension (CTEPH)). These patients do not develop PPA for reasons that are unclear and have different pathophysiology, and therefore require different management strategies.

Pulmonary Hypertension Pathophysiology

The development of PH is multifactorial and complex. It is initiated by different factors according to the underlying disease process. Although PAH occurs in association with diverse aetiologies it results in the distinct pathophysiological process of PPA [3].

Plexogenic Pulmonary Arteriopathy (PPA)

The vascular endothelium normally releases a number of factors that have important roles in the control of vasomotor tone, cellular proliferation and platelet aggregation in the pulmonary circulation. These include nitric oxide, prostacyclin and

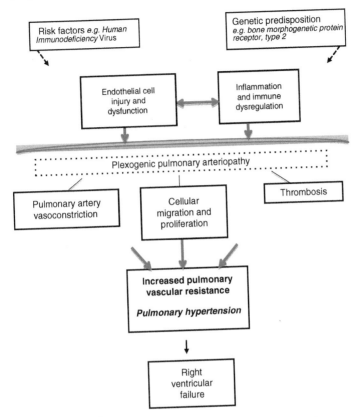

FIGURE 1.1 Factors involved in the pathophysiology of pulmonary arterial hypertension

endothelin and will be detailed in Chap. 2. In PPA, endothelial dysfunction leads to an imbalance in these factors which results in a number of changes that increase PVR (Fig. 1.1):

Vasoconstriction

In accordance with Poiseuille's law the flow of blood through a vessel is proportional to its radius to the fourth power. Consequently, relatively small reductions in vessel radius are accompanied by large reductions in blood flow. For example if the radius of a vessel is halved then blood flow is decreased by a factor of 16. Paralleling Ohm's law relating to electrical principles, PVR is determined by dividing the pressure drop through the pulmonary circulation by total pulmonary blood flow. Therefore a significant fall in blood flow from a reduction in the radius of vessels is associated with a significant increase in PVR.

The endothelial dysfunction in PAH and the imbalance between tissue and circulating vasoactive factors leads to pulmonary arterial vasoconstriction which reduces vessel radius, significantly reduces blood flow and increases PVR [4–6].

Cellular Proliferation and Thrombosis

In the early stages of PPA hypertrophy, recruitment and proliferation of smooth muscle results in thickening of the subendothelial tunica media layer of the distal pulmonary arteries. Activated vascular cells then obtain migratory and invasive properties in addition to hyperproliferative properties. They migrate from the inner half of the tunica media of pulmonary arterioles and travel to the vascular lumen. In the lumen they become myofibroblasts which proliferate and lay down smooth muscle and fibrous tissue in a concentric fashion. This causes vascular narrowing (i.e., a reduction in vessel radius) and/or occlusion and blood flow is significantly reduced according to Poiseuille's law so PVR increases. At points of weakness, especially when the blood vessels are branching, they rupture with subsequent haemorrhage. Disorganised primitive blood vessels grow into these areas and are termed plexiform lesions. The plexiform lesions are composed of multiple cell types including apoptosis-resistant endothelial cells, progenitor cells and immune cells [3, 7].

The endothelial dysfunction and the associated imbalance in endothelium derived vascular mediators gives rise to a hypercoagulable phenotype in PAH [8]. This promotes the development of *in situ* thrombosis. The development of thrombus in the already narrowed pulmonary arteries further obstructs and reduces blood flow, increasing PVR.

Mechanisms of Disease

The exact mechanisms behind the development of PPA are not fully understood. Pulmonary endothelial dysfunction has a central role in its initiation and progression [9–12]. Certain risk factors can facilitate this endothelial damage and dysfunction, including autoimmune diseases, toxins and HIV infection. Inflammation, including cytokines and immune cells appear to play a significant role in the initiation and evolution of PPA [13]. Many factors with roles in normal cell growth and/or angiogenesis are altered to promote cell proliferation and disordered angiogenesis [14–16]. Mitochondrial metabolism in proliferating vascular cells in PPA is shifted from oxidative phosphorylation to glycolysis in the same way as cancer [17].

Sometimes genetic factors confer a predisposition to cellular proliferation and the development of PPA (hereditary PAH). TGF-β signalling generally has a negative effect on cell growth, controlling cell proliferation and apoptosis. The bone morphogenetic type 2 receptor (BMPR2) belongs to the transforming growth factor-beta (TGF-β) superfamily and is expressed in pulmonary vascular smooth muscle and endothelial cells. BMPR2 normally has a protective role, suppressing smooth muscle cell proliferation and normalising endothelial cell apoptosis. Reduced expression or loss of function from mutation of the BMPR2 gene leads to a loss of its growth inhibitory effect and a tendency towards the development of PPA [18]. Genetic predisposition to PPA also occurs less commonly from mutation of downstream mediators (e.g., cytoplasmic signalling proteins- smad proteins) or key regulators (e.g., activin A receptor kinase-1 mutations) in TGF-β signalling [19].

The vascular endothelium, vascular remodelling and inflammatory mechanisms in PAH will be discussed further in Chap. 2.

Pulmonary Veno-occlusive Disease and Pulmonary Capillary Haemangiomatosis

In most conditions associated with PAH the pulmonary veins do not offer a significant contribution to the haemodynamic compromise in the pulmonary circulation and cellular proliferation is not present in the capillary bed. However, this is not the case in pulmonary veno-occlusive disease (PVOD) and pulmonary capillary haemangiomatosis (PCH) which belong to a rare subset of PAH. In PVOD, patients develop significant fibro-occlusive lesions, muscularisation and inflammation of the septal veins and pre-septal venules in addition to a degree of distal pulmonary arteriopathy [20]. In PCH, cellular proliferation arises in the alveolar capillaries. Invasion of adjacent vascular, pulmonary and bronchial structures is typically seen, often associated with diffuse alveolar haemorrhage [21]. Both PCH and PVOD can clinically masquerade as idiopathic PAH but the distinction is extremely important for patient management as pulmonary vasodilators may be deleterious in these patients.

The Pathophysiology of Other Clinical Groups

The development of PPA is reserved to conditions which are classified in the subgroup PAH. Although occlusive lesions and plexiform lesions are exclusive to PPA, endothelial dysfunction leads to pulmonary arterial vasoconstriction, structural remodelling and cellular proliferation in other PH clinical groups. This includes CTEPH [22], PH in the setting of chronic lung disease [23] and left heart disease [24].

Left Heart Disease

Patients classified as having PH secondary to left heart disease (for example left ventricular failure or mitral valve disease) have an elevated left atrial filling pressure which is defined at right heart catheterisation by an elevated pulmonary wedge pressure (PWP >15 mmHg). These patients initially develop a passive rise in mPAP as a consequence of elevated back pressure to the pulmonary circulation from an increase in left atrial filling pressure. This can be associated with a normal or slightly elevated PVR, pulmonary perfusion abnormalities and vascular remodelling. With disease progression, there is superimposed pulmonary vasoconstriction and further vascular remodelling and patients develop established pulmonary vascular disease, associated with significant increases in PVR.

Chronic Lung Disease

Physiological pulmonary vasoconstriction occurs in response to alveolar hypoxia as an important way of matching regional blood flow and alveolar ventilation. In chronic lung disease and or chronic hypoxia, hypoxic vasoconstriction has a key role in PH pathogenesis. However, endothelial dysfunction and inflammation are believed to play the major role in the pathogenesis of PH secondary to chronic lung disease [25].

Chronic Thromboembolic Pulmonary Hypertension

CTEPH is diagnosed when chronically obstructed pulmonary arteries from pulmonary thromboemboli (PE) are associated with pathologically elevated PVR and pulmonary arterial pressure [26]. In this condition, unresolved thrombi become organised and remodel to cause chronic fibrous obstructions within the pulmonary arteries which resists blood flow [27].

The severity of pulmonary artery pressure elevation does not necessarily correlate with the degree of pulmonary vascular obstruction visualised on imaging, nor does the level of PVR necessarily correlate with similar degrees of vascular obstruction associated with acute PE. This is due to progressive distal vasculopathy development in both the occluded

8   J. Bacon and B. Madden

and non-occluded regions [28–31]. Muscular hypertrophy resulting in vasoconstriction and fibrointimal proliferation narrows the lumen of the distal pulmonary arteries [22]. It is therefore both the extent of chronic vascular obstruction from organised thrombi and secondary small vessel arteriopathy that contribute to elevated PVR in CTEPH.

CTEPH appears to develop in only 4 % of patients who have previously been diagnosed with acute PE [32], although 60 % of patients that are diagnosed with CTEPH have never had a clinically apparent acute PE [33, 34]. Mechanisms implicated in the pathogenesis of why some patients develop CTEPH include recurrence of PE, in situ thrombosis, unsuccessful resolution of the initial PE or its propagation into branch pulmonary vessels [35]. Abnormalities in the clotting cascade, platelets and endothelium appear to interact in the coagulation process, initiating or exacerbating the development of thromboemboli and/or *in situ* thrombosis. Some patients have an identifiable abnormality associated with thrombophilia such as protein S or C deficiency or the presence of antiphospholipid antibodies [36].

Pulmonary thromboendarterectomy is the treatment of choice for selected CTEPH patients, offering surgical removal of proximal pulmonary arterial obstruction and therefore potential cure. However, patients with significant distal disease do not benefit from surgery. This will be discussed further in Chap. 4.

Right Ventricular Failure

The pulmonary circulation is normally a low resistance, low pressure network. It can ordinarily accommodate increasing pulmonary blood flow, even during maximal exertion, without a rise in pulmonary arterial pressure. This occurs from passive changes in the compliant pulmonary arteries and capillary beds. Vessels distend and microcirculatory reserves are recruited to lower PVR and to maintain a low pressure circulation [37]. Similarly, early pulmonary vascular disease can be compensated for and is therefore typically subclinical.

The normal low pressure and resistance in the pulmonary circulation offers a low afterload to the right ventricle (RV). It is therefore not adapted to work at high pressure but is adapted to accommodate the variable haemodynamic demands placed upon it. The RV is relatively thin walled and compliant compared with the thick walled left ventricle, but it hypertrophies as the pulmonary artery pressure increases. Initially the RV can overcome the increased afterload associated with a higher PVR [38] but later, cardiomyocyte contractility declines and as the contractile force weakens the RV dilates. RV dilatation increases wall tension and oxygen demand whilst decreasing perfusion. This further decreases contractile function and a vicious cycle ensues [39]. The contractile reserve and the transition from RV hypertrophy to failure is dependent not only on the severity and time course of increasing afterload but also on the degree of oxidative stress, reduced myocardial perfusion, neuro-hormonal and immune activation and the response of the RV to this including remodelling and fibrosis [37, 38, 40–43].

The usual cause of death in patients with PH is RV failure, when increasing PVR causes progressive elevation in afterload which RV contractility can no longer accommodate [28, 44].

Clinical Presentation

PH typically has an insidious onset, with non-specific symptoms. Clinical findings are commonly attributed to concomitant diseases. It is therefore a challenging diagnosis to consider and investigate, especially early in the disease process. Failure to diagnose or incorrect diagnosis is common [45]. A reported median of 14 months from onset of symptoms to diagnosis has been found [46]. A high clinical index of suspicion is necessary, especially in patient groups at increased risk of developing PH.

Symptoms

Patients with early PH may be asymptomatic. The first symptoms that usually develop are fatigue and dyspnoea on exertion. With disease progression symptoms become more apparent, as the PVR escalates and cardiac output falls. Breathlessness with diminishing exertion and then at rest ensues. Palpitations, chest pain (right ventricular angina), presyncopal episodes and later syncope can develop. As the right heart fails, symptoms advance to include peripheral oedema and abdominal swelling from ascites. Eventually, without successful treatment, patients die from RV failure [38, 47, 48].

Functional Classification

Patients with PH are classified according to the World Health Organisation (WHO) 1998 New York Heart Association functional classification (FC). This classifies the patient according to the symptoms they experience during daily living (Table 1.1) [1]. A patient's functional class is important in determining their prognosis and helps determine disease severity and response to treatment.

Physical Examination

Abnormal physical findings may be subtle in patients with PH and can be missed. A loud pulmonary component to the second heart sound may be heard from forceful pulmonary valve closure secondary to elevated pulmonary artery pressure. The jugular venous pressure may depict a prominent 'a' wave from high RV filling pressures. With RV dilatation the tricuspid apparatus can dilate resulting in functional regurgitation and accentuated 'v' waves identifiable in the jugular venous waveform. Equally the pansystolic murmur of

TABLE 1.1 Functional classification of patients with pulmonary hypertension according to the World Health Organisation, modified after the New York Heart Association functional classification [1]

Class	Description
I	Patients with pulmonary hypertension but without resulting limitation of physical activity. Ordinary physical activity does not cause undue dyspnoea or fatigue, chest pain, or near syncope.
II	Patients with pulmonary hypertension resulting in slight limitation of physical activity. They are comfortable at rest. Ordinary physical activity causes undue dyspnoea or fatigue, chest pain, or near syncope.
III	Patients with pulmonary hypertension resulting in marked limitation of physical activity. They are comfortable at rest. Less than ordinary activity causes undue dyspnoea or fatigue, chest pain, or near syncope.
IV	Patients with pulmonary hypertension with inability to carry out any physical activity without symptoms. These patients manifest signs of right heart failure. Dyspnoea and/or fatigue may even be present at rest. Discomfort is increased by any physical activity.

tricuspid regurgitation may be audible. A left parasternal lift can occur as a consequence of RV hypertrophy. A right ventricular fourth heart sound (immediately prior to the first heart sound) may result from abnormal turbulent blood flow as the right atrium contracts and forces blood flow into a stiffened RV. Alternatively with RV dysfunction and volume overload a third heart sound may follow the second heart sound in mid diastole during ventricular filling. With RV failure, jugular venous distension, hepatomegaly, ascites and peripheral oedema are common features. Arrhythmia may develop as a consequence of atrial dilatation or RV dilatation, hypertrophy or fibrosis and rhythm disturbance is important to recognise on clinical examination as it can impede cardiac function.

Diagnosis

PH is defined by the resting mPAP measured at right heart catheterisation (>=25 mmHg). Therefore, the diagnosis of PH ordinarily requires invasive confirmation.

The normal value of mPAP is 14 ± 3 mmHg [1, 49]. Patients with borderline mPAP values (17–24 mmHg) should be prospectively monitored for the development of PH and research into the significance and suitable management of these patients is ongoing.

Right Heart Catheterisation

Right heart catheterisation (Fig. 1.2) measures the pressure, flow and resistance in the cardiopulmonary circulation, including measurement of the downstream left atrial pressure (PWP). Cardiac shunting can also be identified and measured by oxygen saturation assessment [50].

PWP is determined by wedging the tip of the right heart catheter with the balloon inflated in the pulmonary artery. The forward flow of blood is temporarily stopped within the small vessel where the catheter lies. When there is no venous obstruction, the measured pressure is the back pressure transmitted from the left atrium, as there are no anatomical valves in the pulmonary veins [51, 52]. A PWP of greater than 15 mmHg defines a significant contribution to raised mPAP from pressure beyond the pulmonary capillary bed, for example from left atrial hypertension.

In general the PWP is not greater than 15 mmHg in patients with PAH [53]. However, the size, shape and compliance of one ventricle has a direct effect on the other ventricle through their mechanical interaction, including a shared septum, myofibres and a joint pericardial space encased by a fibrous pericardium. Therefore, left ventricular dysfunction can result from significant RV dysfunction, and this can lead to elevated left atrial filling pressure and PWP in PAH [54].

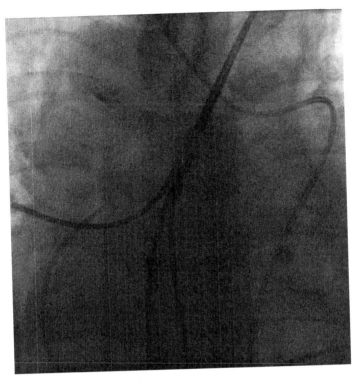

FIGURE 1.2 Plain radiograph showing a right heart catheter in the pulmonary artery of a patient with dextrocardia (precordial leads also shown)

PWP may also be elevated (or normal) in pulmonary veno-occlusive disease. This depends on the size of the veins involved and the degree of collateral communication between the affected venous beds [20].

Ohm's law pertaining to electrical resistance states that resistance equals pressure divided by flow. Therefore, PVR is calculated by dividing the transpulmonary pressure gradient (mPAP – PWP (mmHg)) by cardiac output (L/min). This is an important measurement determined by right heart catheterisation which is commonly measured in arbitrary units called

Wood Units (WU). One Wood Unit is 1 mmHg per litre per minute or 80 dynes.sec.cm^{-5} [55]. PVR is abnormal when above 2WU but is defined as significantly raised when greater than 3WU [53, 56, 57]. A pathological elevation in PVR signifies the presence of significant pulmonary vasculopathy. PVR greater than 3WU is included in the definition of PAH [53].

Right heart catheterisation identifies important prognostic variables for patients with PH. Mean right atrial pressure, cardiac index (cardiac output adjusted for body surface area) and PVR have been shown to predict mortality in national PAH registries [58–60]. Notably PVR is a more important variable than mPAP in the assessment of the severity and prognosis of PH [61]. Progressive pulmonary vasculopathy is translated into an increasing PVR. Paradoxically, with increasing afterload the RV starts to fail and the cardiac output reduces, and this can result in a fall of mPAP despite advancing disease.

Right heart catheterisation procedures are generally well tolerated [62] but due to their invasive nature significant serious adverse events (1.1 %) and mortality (0.1 %) have been reported in multicentre large patient series [63]. However, right heart catheterisation accurately defines an individual's pulmonary haemodynamics to establish a diagnosis of PH. It aids treatment decisions including suggesting contributing factors, identifying important prognostic variables and assessing disease progression.

Non invasive Investigations

Although right heart catheterisation is the gold standard diagnostic investigation for PH, non invasive estimates are advantageous in terms of cost, availability and risk. They are used to help identify those patients that require further investigation into a diagnosis of PH but they cannot reliably exclude the diagnosis. Non invasive investigations are important in establishing conditions causing or contributing to the diagnosis of PH such as thromboemboli, left heart or lung disease.

Echocardiography

Echocardiography is used to aid the diagnosis of PH initially, risk-stratify patients and monitor their progress. It is also important in the identification of valvular pathology, cardiac shunts (especially when contrast is used) and primary myocardial disease, that may contribute to a diagnosis of PH [64].

Transthoracic echocardiography determines the pulmonary arterial pressure to aid the identification and monitoring of PH patients. The most common method is determining the pulmonary artery systolic pressure by the velocity of measurable tricuspid regurgitation (Fig. 1.3). A meta-analysis of this method revealed a moderate diagnostic accuracy of 83 % sensitivity (95 % confidence interval 73–90 %) and 72 % specificity (95 % confidence interval 53–85 %) when compared to invasive measurement [65]. The wide confidence intervals highlight the weakness of echocardiography as a sole investigative or screening tool in PH.

Increasing afterload in PH stresses the thin walled and distensible right ventricle to forge its shape, size and functional state. When adequate echocardiography views are obtained, the morphology and function of the RV can be assessed to serially evaluate RV dysfunction and suggest the presence of PH. In addition, the discussed interaction between the right and left ventricle can be visualised, and the size and pressure within the right atrium can be reviewed. The presence of a pericardial effusion can be established easily by echocardiography which has been shown to predict death or transplantation in PAH [66, 67].

As PH cannot reliably be defined by a cut off pulmonary artery pressure value using echocardiography alone, current guidelines suggest incorporating other echocardiography measures and determining the probability of PH. PH is unlikely in the presence of pulmonary artery systolic pressures below 36 mmHg in the absence of additional echocardiogram variables suggestive of PH, possible at higher values and likely when greater than 50 mmHg (Table 1.2) [1, 49]. It

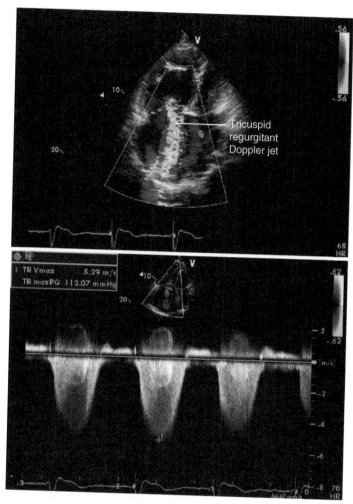

FIGURE 1.3 Pulmonary artery systolic pressure estimation by the continuous wave Doppler tracing of the tricuspid regurgitant jet velocity in a patient with pulmonary hypertension. From a tricuspid regurgitant velocity of 5.29 m/s the right ventricular systolic pressure can be calculated to 135–140 mmHg, equivalent to pulmonary artery systolic pressure in the absence of right ventricular outflow obstruction

TABLE 1.2 Arbitrary criteria for estimating the presence of pulmonary hypertension (PH) by echocardiography, according to international guidelines [1]

Echocardiography diagnosis of PH	Tricuspid regurgitant peak velocity	Pulmonary artery systolic pressure*	Additional echocardiogram variables suggestive of PH
Unlikely	≤2.8 m/s	≤36 mmHg	No
Possible	≤2.8 m/s	≤36 mmHg	Yes
Possible	2.9–3.4 m/s	37–50 mmHg	Yes/no
Likely	>3.4 m/s	>50 mmHg	Yes/no

*assuming a normal right atrial pressure of 5 mmHg

is essential that the full diagnostic potential of echocardiography is used when assessing PH.

Other Routine Investigations

An electrocardiogram is important in PH to identify and diagnose arrhythmia so that suitable management can be initiated. The electrocardiogram may also show evidence of right atrial enlargement, right ventricular strain or hypertrophy [68] to suggest a diagnosis of PH. However, it is not a sufficient screening tool for the presence of PH, especially in early disease [47].

At present, the place for radiological investigation in patients with suspected PH is mainly in the identification of lung diseases or CTEPH. However, recognition of pulmonary artery enlargement or dilatation of cardiac chambers from imaging can suggest the diagnosis of PH (Fig. 1.4).

A baseline chest radiograph is considered routine and may reveal features suggestive of PH, left ventricular impairment (Table 1.3), or lung disease.

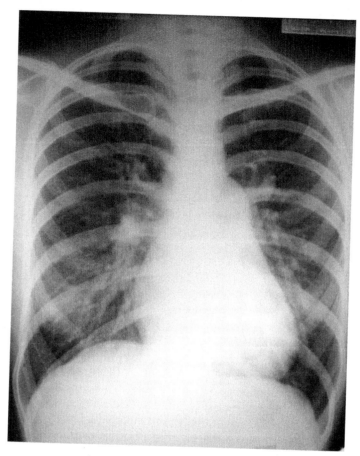

FIGURE 1.4 Chest radiograph showing plethoric pulmonary arterial vasculature with right ventricular enlargement elevating the cardiac apex and reduced size of the aortic knuckle in a patient with pulmonary hypertension from atrial septal defect

Computed tomography (CT) offers a simultaneous assessment of the pulmonary vasculature (pulmonary angiography) and lung parenchyma (high resolution CT) and is the main diagnostic strategy in PH radiological investigation (Fig. 1.5)

TABLE 1.3 Chest radiograph features suggestive of left ventricular impairment

Chest radiograph feature	Stage of left ventricular impairment progression
Cardiac enlargement	Variable, widely prevalent in chronic cases
Upper lobe venous redistribution	Elevated pulmonary venous pressure
Central venous prominence	Elevated pulmonary venous pressure
Indistinctness of the central perihilar vasculature	Interstitial oedema
Thickening of the minor fissure	Interstitial oedema
Pleural effusion	Interstitial oedema
Diffuse air space disease	Alveolar oedema

[69, 70]. The presence of acute or chronic thromboembolic disease related to CTEPH or lung diseases such as emphysema can be recognised by CT. CT imaging can also be helpful in identifying PVOD and PCH which are typically challenging to diagnose. PVOD typically demonstrates features of pulmonary interstitial oedema without engorgement of the main pulmonary veins or left sided chambers (as the occlusion is in the more proximal post capillary venules). Comparatively, extensive ground glass nodules are typical in PCH [71].

Ventilation perfusion scintigraphy is used to further investigate the presence of CTEPH by identifying the mismatch between perfusion and ventilation from vessel occlusion [72, 73].

Pulmonary function testing is performed to identify lung disease as a contributor to PH. With adequate technique, physiological impairment from underlying respiratory disease can be identified and quantified. However, even without concomitant lung disease, a reduction in carbon monoxide diffusion is typically demonstrated in PAH. Damage to the pulmonary vascular bed in PAH results in decreased capillary

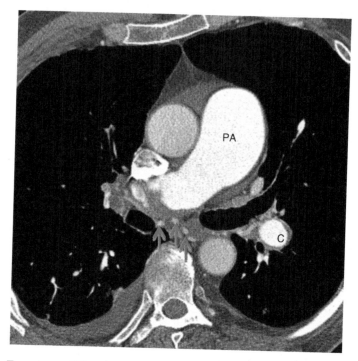

FIGURE 1.5 CT pulmonary angiogram showing bronchial artery hypertrophy (*arrows*) in a patient with chronic thromboembolic pulmonary hypertension. Note the marked enlargement of the pulmonary artery (*PA*) and the rim of clot around the left lower lobe pulmonary artery (*C*)

blood volume and flow and a reduction in the surface area available for gas diffusion [74, 75]. An unexpected reduction in a patient's gas diffusion should guide the physician to consider a diagnosis of PAH.

Routine haematological and biochemical investigations in PH include full blood count, urea and electrolytes and liver function testing. Liver function testing is important to recognise a predisposition to and potential cause of PH, with consideration given to liver ultrasound. Similarly, autoimmune profiles may help identify underlying connective tissue diseases, and HIV testing in patients with PH is recommended [1]. Screening for thrombophilia or sickle cell disease is appropriate in patients with a suggestive history. Genetic testing is important in idiopathic and heritable PAH including the offer of genetic counselling and testing of relatives.

Brain natriuretic peptide (BNP) and the biologically inactive N-terminal segment (NT-proBNP) can be measured in the blood and are released from the myocardium in response to wall stress. In the presence of right ventricular dysfunction these markers typically rise and therefore they are useful for monitoring disease progression in PH. An elevated or increasing level of BNP or NT-proBNP is a poor prognostic sign suggesting progressive right ventricular dysfunction [76]. However, in early disease before significant cardiac dysfunction, their levels can be normal and their levels will also rise in response to left ventricular dysfunction. An elevation in BNP or NT-pro BNP level is therefore not specific to a diagnosis of PH nor does a normal level exclude the condition [77, 78].

Six Minute Walk Distance

The six minute walk test measures the distance a patient can walk on the flat in a 6 min period without encouragement. It is easily carried out, inexpensive and the results correlate well with functional status [79]. Patients may be used as their own control, to monitor their response to treatment.

A patient's six minute walk distance has historically been used as a common clinical trial end point in PH. However, a patient's six minute walk distance is not necessarily a reliable marker of pulmonary vascular disease progression or improvement as it is a nonspecific general exercise capacity test [80]. Results depend not only on the severity of PH but also are highly dependent on simple demographic characteristics, co-morbidities of the patient and other day to day variables. A meta-analysis by Savarese et al. reviewed 22 clinical trials using six minute walk testing to assess pharmacological treatments. Although favourable effects on clinical events were present such as reduced all-cause mortality, these were not predicted by change in six minute walk distance [81]. Recent drug trials in PH have moved away from change in six minute walk distance and towards time to 'clinical worsening' as a more suitable primary trial endpoint for these reasons [82].

Disease Classification

Once identified, the separate conditions that predispose and or cause PH are used to classify patients into distinct groups according to common pathological and clinical features (Table 1.4) [83, 84]. PAH is classified as group 1, PH associated with left heart diseases are classified as group 2, PH associated with lung diseases and or hypoxia are in group 3, CTEPH belongs in group 4 and group 5 includes diseases with unclear multifactorial mechanisms such as sarcoidosis or sickle cell disease.

PAH has an estimated prevalence of 15–26 cases/million [85]. This likely represents approximately 10 % of all PH patients [86]. No precise estimates for the more prevalent subtypes of PH including groups 2 and 3 are available however they are recognised as major health burdens [25].

Of the diseases associated with PAH, the estimated life time risk of PH in patients with congenital heart disease is 4–15 % [87]; 5–12 % in systemic sclerosis [88]; 0.5–10 % in portal hypertension [89] and 0.5 % in HIV [90]. Those patients that are genetic carriers of the BMPR2 mutation have a 20 % increased life time risk of PAH development [91]. Patients with sickle cell disease have a 2–3.7 % risk of developing pulmonary vasculopathy [92–94].

Survival

The median survival for patients with PAH is 2.8 years when untreated [45]. Unfortunately even with modern management PAH remains a progressive and fatal disease, with 1 year

TABLE 1.4 The classification of pulmonary hypertension according to the World Congress, Nice 2013

Group	Subtypes	Clinical examples
Group 1: Pulmonary Arterial Hypertension	Idiopathic	
	Heritable	BMPR2, ALK-1, ENH, SMAD9, CAV1, KCNK3
	Drug/toxin induced	Anorexigens, metamphetamines
	Conditions associated with pulmonary arterial hypertension	Connective tissue disease
		Congenital heart diseases
		Portal hypertension
		Human immunodeficiency virus infection
		Schistosomiasis
Group 1'	Pulmonary veno-occlusive disease and or Pulmonary capillary haemangiomatosis	

(continued)

TABLE 1.4 (continued)

Group	Subtypes	Clinical examples
Group 2: Pulmonary hypertension due to left heart disease	Left ventricular systolic dysfunction	
	Left ventricular diasystolic dysfunction	
	Valvular disease	
Group 3: Pulmonary hypertension due to lung diseases and/or hypoxia	Chronic obstructive pulmonary disease	
	Interstitial lung disease	
	Other pulmonary diseases with mixed obstructive and restrictive pattern	
	Sleep disordered breathing and alveolar hypoventilation disorders	Obstructive sleep apnoea, obesity hypoventilation, neuromuscular disorders
	Chronic exposure to high altitude	
	Developmental lung diseases	

Group 4: Chronic thromboembolic pulmonary hypertension		
Group 5: Pulmonary hypertension with unclear multifactorial mechanisms	Haematological disorders	Myeloproliferative disorders, splenectomy, **chronic haemolytic anaemia**[*]
	Systemic disorders	Sarcoidosis, lymphamgioleiomatosis
	Metabolic disorders	Glycogen storage disease
		Thyroid disorders
	Others	Chronic renal failure

The main change made from the Dana point 2008 World Congress is highlighted (*)
BMPR2 bone morphogenic protein receptor type 2, *CAV1-1* caveolin-1, *ENG* endoglin, *ALK-1* ativin-like receptor kinase-1, *KCNK3* potassium channel super family K member −3, *SMAD 9* mothers against decantaplegic 9

[*]Reclassified from Group 1 to Group 5 at the World Symposium on Pulmonary Hypertension, Nice 2013

incident mortality of 15 % [95] and 55–73 % 3 year survival reported [59, 96]. However, studies on PAH treatment suggest that the earlier that disease modifying therapies are implemented, the better the outcome for patients [89].

Key Learning Points

- Pulmonary hypertension is defined as resting mean pulmonary artery pressure (mPAP)>=25 mmHg.
- Right heart catheterisation is the gold standard diagnostic investigation in PH
- Pulmonary wedge pressure (PWP) approximates left atrial filling pressure.
- Pulmonary vascular resistance (PVR)

$$\left(\text{Wood Units}\right) = \frac{\text{mPAP} - \text{PWP}\left(\text{mmHg}\right)}{\text{Cardiac output}\left(\text{L / min}\right)}$$

- Noninvasive investigations help define the probability of the presence of PH and identify causes or contributors to the diagnosis.
- Conditions classified in Group 1 pulmonary arterial hypertension have similar pathophysiology termed plexogenic pulmonary arteriopathy and therefore distinct management.
- Pulmonary hypertension is a progressive and ultimately fatal disease without appropriate treatment. In the presence of increasing PVR the right ventricle ultimately fails.

References

1. Galie N, Hoeper MM, Humbert M, Torbicki A, Vachiery JL, Barbera JA, Beghetti M, Corris P, Gaine S, Gibbs JS, Gomez-Sanchez MA, Jondeau G, Klepetko W, Opitz C, Peacock A, Rubin L, Zellweger M, Simonneau G, ESC Committee for Practice Guidelines (CPG). Guidelines for the diagnosis and treatment of pulmonary hypertension: the Task Force for the Diagnosis and Treatment of Pulmonary Hypertension of the

European Society of Cardiology (ESC) and the European Respiratory Society (ERS), endorsed by the International Society of Heart and Lung Transplantation (ISHLT). Eur Heart J. 2009;30(20):2493–537.

2. Madden B, Gosney J, Coghlan J, Kamalvand K, Caslin A, Smith P, et al. Pretransplant clinicopathological correlation in end-stage primary pulmonary hypertension. Eur Respir J. 1994;7(4):672–8.

3. Smith P, Heath D, Yacoub M, Madden B, Caslin A, Gosney J. The ultrastructure of plexogenic pulmonary arteriopathy. J Pathol. 1990;160(2):111–21.

4. MacLean MR. Endothelin-1: a mediator of pulmonary hypertension? Pulm Pharmacol Ther. 1998;11(2–3):125–32.

5. Moncada S, Palmer RM, Higgs EA. Nitric oxide: physiology, pathophysiology, and pharmacology. Pharmacol Rev. 1991;43(2): 109–42.

6. Tuder RM, Cool CD, Geraci MW, Wang J, Abman SH, Wright L, et al. Prostacyclin synthase expression is decreased in lungs from patients with severe pulmonary hypertension. Am J Respir Crit Care Med. 1999;159(6):1925–32.

7. Heath D, Smith P, Gosney J. The pathology of the early and late stages of primary pulmonary hypertension. Br Heart J. 1987;58(3): 204–13.

8. Tournier A, Wahl D, Chaouat A, Max J, Regnault V, Lecompte T, et al. Calibrated automated thrombography demonstrates hyper-coagulability in patients with idiopathic pulmonary arterial hypertension. Thromb Res. 2010;126(6):e418–22.

9. Eddahibi S, Guignabert C, Barlier-Mur AM, Dewachter L, Fadel E, Dartevelle P, et al. Cross talk between endothelial and smooth muscle cells in pulmonary hypertension: critical role for serotonin-induced smooth muscle hyperplasia. Circulation. 2006;113(15):1857–64.

10. Davie N, Haleen SJ, Upton PD, Polak JM, Yacoub MH, Morrell NW, et al. ET(A) and ET(B) receptors modulate the proliferation of human pulmonary artery smooth muscle cells. Am J Respir Crit Care Med. 2002;165(3):398–405.

11. Burg ED, Remillard CV, Yuan JX. Potassium channels in the regulation of pulmonary artery smooth muscle cell proliferation and apoptosis: pharmacotherapeutic implications. Br J Pharmacol. 2008;153 Suppl 1:S99–111.

12. Toshner M, Voswinckel R, Southwood M, Al-Lamki R, Howard LS, Marchesan D, et al. Evidence of dysfunction of endothelial

progenitors in pulmonary arterial hypertension. Am J Respir Crit Care Med. 2009;180(8):780–7.

13. Hassoun PM, Mouthon L, Barbera JA, Eddahibi S, Flores SC, Grimminger F, et al. Inflammation, growth factors, and pulmonary vascular remodeling. J Am Coll Cardiol. 2009;54(1 Suppl):S10–9.

14. Ameshima S, Golpon H, Cool CD, Chan D, Vandivier RW, Gardai SJ, et al. Peroxisome proliferator-activated receptor gamma (PPARgamma) expression is decreased in pulmonary hypertension and affects endothelial cell growth. Circ Res. 2003;92(10):1162–9.

15. Li X, Zhang X, Leathers R, Makino A, Huang C, Parsa P, et al. Notch3 signaling promotes the development of pulmonary arterial hypertension. Nat Med. 2009;15(11):1289–97.

16. Chelladurai P, Seeger W, Pullamsetti SS. Matrix metalloproteinases and their inhibitors in pulmonary hypertension. Eur Respir J. 2012;40(3):766–82.

17. Bonnet S, Michelakis ED, Porter CJ, Andrade-Navarro MA, Thebaud B, Bonnet S, et al. An abnormal mitochondrial-hypoxia inducible factor-1alpha-Kv channel pathway disrupts oxygen sensing and triggers pulmonary arterial hypertension in fawn hooded rats: similarities to human pulmonary arterial hypertension. Circulation. 2006;113(22):2630–41.

18. Newman JH, Wheeler L, Lane KB, Loyd E, Gaddipati R, Phillips 3rd JA, et al. Mutation in the gene for bone morphogenetic protein receptor II as a cause of primary pulmonary hypertension in a large kindred. N Engl J Med. 2001;345(5):319–24.

19. Morrell NW. Pulmonary hypertension due to BMPR2 mutation: a new paradigm for tissue remodelling? Proc Am Thorac Soc. 2006;3:680–6.

20. Harris P, Heath D. Pulmonary veno-occlusive disease human pulmonary circulation. 3rd ed. New York: Churchill; 1986. p. 74–6.

21. Wagenvoort CA, Beetstra A, Spijker J. Capillary haemangiomatosis of the lungs. Histopathology. 1978;2(6):401–6.

22. Jamieson SW, Kapelanski DP. Pulmonary endarterectomy. Curr Probl Surg. 2000;37(3):165–252.

23. Wilkinson M, Langhorne CA, Heath D, Barer GR, Howard P. A pathophysiological study of 10 cases of hypoxic cor pulmonale. Q J Med. 1988;66(249):65–85.

24. Delgado JF, Conde E, Sanchez V, Lopez-Rios F, Gomez-Sanchez MA, Escribano P, et al. Pulmonary vascular remodeling in pulmonary hypertension due to chronic heart failure. Eur J Heart Fail. 2005;7(6):1011–6.

25. Lourenco AP, Fontoura D, Henriques-Coelho T, Leite-Moreira AF. Current pathophysiological concepts and management of pulmonary hypertension. Int J Cardiol. 2012;155(3):350–61.
26. Jenkins D, Mayer E, Screaton N, Madani M. State-of-the-art chronic thromboembolic pulmonary hypertension diagnosis and management. Eur Respir Rev. 2012;21(123):32–9.
27. Keogh AM, Mayer E, Benza RL, Corris P, Dartevelle PG, Frost AE, et al. Interventional and surgical modalities of treatment in pulmonary hypertension. J Am Coll Cardiol. 2009;54(1 Suppl):S67–77.
28. Humbert M. Pulmonary arterial hypertension and chronic thromboembolic pulmonary hypertension: pathophysiology. Eur Respir Rev. 2010;19(115):59–63.
29. Delcroix M, Vonk Noordegraaf A, Fadel E, Lang I, Simonneau G, Naeije R. Vascular and right ventricular remodelling in chronic thromboembolic pulmonary hypertension. Eur Respir J. 2013;41(1):224–32.
30. Moser KM, Bloor CM. Pulmonary vascular lesions occurring in patients with chronic major vessel thromboembolic pulmonary hypertension. Chest. 1993;103(3):685–92.
31. Sage E, Mercier O, Herve P, Tu L, Dartevelle P, Eddahibi S, et al. Right lung ischemia induces contralateral pulmonary vasculopathy in an animal model. J Thorac Cardiovasc Surg. 2012;143(4):967–73.
32. Pengo V, Lensing AW, Prins MH, Marchiori A, Davidson BL, Tiozzo F, et al. Incidence of chronic thromboembolic pulmonary hypertension after pulmonary embolism. N Engl J Med. 2004;350(22):2257–64.
33. Condliffe R, Kiely DG, Gibbs JSR, Corris PA, Peacock AJ, Jenkins DP, et al. Prognostic and aetiological factors in chronic thromboembolic pulmonary hypertension. Eur Respir J. 2009;33(2):332–8.
34. Bonderman D, Wilkens H, Wakounig S, Schäfers H, Jansa P, Lindner J, et al. Risk factors for chronic thromboembolic pulmonary hypertension. Eur Respir J. 2009;33(2):325–31.
35. Tuder RM, Abman SH, Braun T, Capron F, Stevens T, Thistlethwaite PA, et al. Development and pathology of pulmonary hypertension. J Am Coll Cardiol. 2009;54(1 Suppl):S3–9.
36. Wolf M, Boyer-Neumann C, Parent F, Eschwege V, Jaillet H, Meyer D, et al. Thrombotic risk factors in pulmonary hypertension. Eur Respir J. 2000;15(2):395–9.
37. Segers VF, Brutsaert DL, De Keulenaer GW. Pulmonary hypertension and right heart failure in heart failure with preserved left

ventricular ejection fraction: pathophysiology and natural history. Curr Opin Cardiol. 2012;27(3):273–80.

38. Bogaard HJ, Abe K, Vonk Noordegraaf A, Voelkel NF. The right ventricle under pressure: cellular and molecular mechanisms of right-heart failure in pulmonary hypertension. Chest. 2009;135(3):794–804.

39. Voelkel NF, Quaife RA, Leinwand LA, Barst RJ, McGoon MD, Meldrum DR, Dupuis J, Long CS, Rubin LJ, Smart FW, Suzuki YJ, Gladwin M, Denholm EM, Gail DB, National Heart, Lung, and Blood Institute Working Group on Cellular and Molecular Mechanisms of Right Heart Failure. Right ventricular function and failure: report of a National Heart, Lung, and Blood Institute working group on cellular and molecular mechanisms of right heart failure. Circulation. 2006;114(17):1883–91.

40. Faber MJ, Dalinghaus M, Lankhuizen IM, Steendijk P, Hop WC, Schoemaker RG, et al. Right and left ventricular function after chronic pulmonary artery banding in rats assessed with biventricular pressure-volume loops. Am J Physiol Heart Circ Physiol. 2006;291(4):H1580–6.

41. Taraseviciene-Stewart L, Kasahara Y, Alger L, Hirth P, Mc Mahon G, Waltenberger J, et al. Inhibition of the VEGF receptor 2 combined with chronic hypoxia causes cell death-dependent pulmonary endothelial cell proliferation and severe pulmonary hypertension. FASEB J. 2001;15(2):427–38.

42. Di Salvo TG. Pulmonary hypertension and right ventricular failure in left ventricular systolic dysfunction. Curr Opin Cardiol. 2012;27(3):262–72.

43. Haddad F, Vrtovec B, Ashley EA, Deschamps A, Haddad H, Denault AY. The concept of ventricular reserve in heart failure and pulmonary hypertension: an old metric that brings us one step closer in our quest for prediction. Curr Opin Cardiol. 2011;26(2):123–31.

44. Voelkel NF, Gomez-Arroyo J, Abbate A, Bogaard HJ, Nicolls MR. Pathobiology of pulmonary arterial hypertension and right ventricular failure. Eur Respir J. 2012;40(6):1555–65.

45. McCann C, Gopalan D, Sheares K, Screaton N. Imaging in pulmonary hypertension, part 1: clinical perspectives, classification, imaging techniques and imaging algorithm. Postgrad Med J. 2012;88(1039):271–9.

46. Pepke-Zaba J, Delcroix M, Lang I, Mayer E, Jansa P, Ambroz D, et al. Chronic thromboembolic pulmonary hypertension (CTEPH): results from an international prospective registry. Circulation. 2011;124(18):1973–81.

47. Rich S, Dantzker DR, Ayres SM. Primary pulmonary hypertension. A national prospective study. Ann Intern Med. 1987;107(2):216–23.

48. Howard LS, Grapsa J, Dawson D, Bellamy M, Chambers JB, Masani ND, et al. Echocardiographic assessment of pulmonary hypertension: standard operating procedure. Eur Respir Rev. 2012;21(125):239–48.

49. Kovacs G, Berghold A, Scheidl S, Olschewski H. Pulmonary arterial pressure during rest and exercise in healthy subjects: a systematic review. Eur Respir J. 2009;34(4):888–94.

50. Guillinta P, Peterson KL, Ben-Yehuda O. Cardiac catheterization techniques in pulmonary hypertension. Cardiol Clin. 2004;22(3):401–15, vi.

51. Lange RA, Moore Jr DM, Cigarroa RG, Hillis LD. Use of pulmonary capillary wedge pressure to assess severity of mitral stenosis: is true left atrial pressure needed in this condition? J Am Coll Cardiol. 1989;13(4):825–31.

52. Connolly DC, Kirklin JW, Wood EH. The relationship between pulmonary artery wedge pressure and left atrial pressure in man. Circ Res. 1954;2(5):434–40.

53. Hoeper MM, Bogaard HJ, Condliffe R, Frantz R, Khanna D, Kurzyna M, et al. Definitions and diagnosis of pulmonary hypertension. J Am Coll Cardiol. 2013;62(25 Suppl):D42–50.

54. Bacon JL, Peerbhoy MS, Wong E, Sharma R, Vlahos I, Crerar-Gilbert A, et al. Current diagnostic investigation in pulmonary hypertension. Curr Respir Med Rev. 2013;9(2):79–100.

55. Chemla D, Castelain V, Hervé P, Lecarpentier Y, Brimioulle S. Haemodynamic evaluation of pulmonary hypertension. Eur Respir J. 2002;20(5):1314–31.

56. Frantz RP. Hemodynamic monitoring in pulmonary arterial hypertension. Expert Rev Respir Med. 2011;5(2):173–8.

57. Gupta H, Ghimire G, Naeije R. The value of tools to assess pulmonary arterial hypertension. Eur Respir Rev. 2011;20(122):222–35.

58. Benza RL, Miller DP, Gomberg-Maitland M, Frantz RP, Foreman AJ, Coffey CS, et al. Predicting survival in pulmonary arterial hypertension: insights from the Registry to Evaluate Early and Long-Term Pulmonary Arterial Hypertension Disease Management (REVEAL). Circulation. 2010;122(2):164–72.

59. Humbert M, Sitbon O, Chaouat A, Bertocchi M, Habib G, Gressin V, et al. Survival in patients with idiopathic, familial, and anorexigen-associated pulmonary arterial hypertension in the modern management era. Circulation. 2010;122(2):156–63.

60. Lee WN, Ling Y, Sheares KK, Pepke-Zaba J, Peacock AJ, Johnson MK. Predicting survival in pulmonary arterial hypertension in the UK. Eur Respir J. 2012;40(3):604–11.
61. Saggar R, Sitbon O. Hemodynamics in pulmonary arterial hypertension: current and future perspectives. Am J Cardiol. 2012;110(6 Suppl):9S–15.
62. Aul R, Bacon J, Anwar M, Fiorino G, Madden B. Right heart catheterization: emerging indications and applications in the optimal management of left heart disease. Am J Respir Crit Care Med. 2013;187:10.1164/ajrccm-conference.2013.187.1_MeetingAbstracts.A4686.
63. Hoeper MM, Lee SH, Voswinckel R, Palazzini M, Jais X, Marinelli A, et al. Complications of right heart catheterization procedures in patients with pulmonary hypertension in experienced centers. J Am Coll Cardiol. 2006;48(12):2546–52.
64. Forfia PR, Vachiery JL. Echocardiography in pulmonary arterial hypertension. Am J Cardiol. 2012;110(6 Suppl):16S–24.
65. Janda S, Shahidi N, Gin K, Swiston J. Diagnostic accuracy of echocardiography for pulmonary hypertension: a systematic review and meta-analysis. Heart. 2011;97(8):612–22.
66. Hinderliter AL, Willis 4th PW, Long W, Clarke WR, Ralph D, Caldwell EJ, et al. Frequency and prognostic significance of pericardial effusion in primary pulmonary hypertension. PPH Study Group. Primary pulmonary hypertension. Am J Cardiol. 1999;84(4):481–4, A10.
67. Raymond RJ, Hinderliter AL, Willis PW, Ralph D, Caldwell EJ, Williams W, et al. Echocardiographic predictors of adverse outcomes in primary pulmonary hypertension. J Am Coll Cardiol. 2002;39(7):1214–9.
68. Bossone E, Paciocco G, Iarussi D, Agretto A, Iacono A, Gillespie BW, et al. The prognostic role of the ECG in primary pulmonary hypertension. Chest. 2002;121(2):513–8.
69. Tsai IC, Tsai WL, Wang KY, Chen MC, Liang KW, Tsai HY, et al. Comprehensive MDCT evaluation of patients with pulmonary hypertension: diagnosing underlying causes with the updated Dana Point 2008 classification. AJR Am J Roentgenol. 2011;197(3):W471–81.
70. Devaraj A, Wells AU, Meister MG, Corte TJ, Hansell DM. The effect of diffuse pulmonary fibrosis on the reliability of CT signs of pulmonary hypertension. Radiology. 2008;249(3):1042–9.
71. Gunther S, Jais X, Maitre S, Berezne A, Dorfmuller P, Seferian A, et al. Computed tomography findings of pulmonary venoocclusive

disease in scleroderma patients presenting with precapillary pulmonary hypertension. Arthritis Rheum. 2012;64(9): 2995–3005.

72. Soler X, Kerr KM, Marsh JJ, Renner JW, Hoh CK, Test VJ, et al. Pilot study comparing SPECT perfusion scintigraphy with CT pulmonary angiography in chronic thromboembolic pulmonary hypertension. Respirology. 2012;17(1):180–4.

73. Tunariu N, Gibbs SJ, Win Z, Gin-Sing W, Graham A, Gishen P, et al. Ventilation-perfusion scintigraphy is more sensitive than multidetector CTPA in detecting chronic thromboembolic pulmonary disease as a treatable cause of pulmonary hypertension. J Nucl Med. 2007;48(5):680–4.

74. Pande JN, Gupta SP, Guleria JS. Clinical significance of the measurement of membrane diffusing capacity and pulmonary cappillary blood volume. Respiration. 1975;32(5):317–24.

75. Steenhuis LH, Groen HJ, Koeter GH, van der Mark TW. Diffusion capacity and haemodynamics in primary and chronic thromboembolic pulmonary hypertension. Eur Respir J. 2000;16(2): 276–81.

76. Nagaya N, Nishikimi T, Uematsu M, Satoh T, Kyotani S, Sakamaki F, et al. Plasma brain natriuretic peptide as a prognostic indicator in patients with primary pulmonary hypertension. Circulation. 2000;102(8):865–70.

77. Mukerjee D, Yap LB, Holmes AM, Nair D, Ayrton P, Black CM, et al. Significance of plasma N-terminal pro-brain natriuretic peptide in patients with systemic sclerosis-related pulmonary arterial hypertension. Respir Med. 2003;97(11):1230–6.

78. Williams MH, Handler CE, Akram R, Smith CJ, Das C, Smee J, et al. Role of N-terminal brain natriuretic peptide (N-TproBNP) in scleroderma-associated pulmonary arterial hypertension. Eur Heart J. 2006;27(12):1485–94.

79. McLaughlin VV, Badesch DB, Delcroix M, Fleming TR, Gaine SP, Galie N, et al. End points and clinical trial design in pulmonary arterial hypertension. J Am Coll Cardiol. 2009;54(1 Suppl):S97–107.

80. McLaughlin VV, Archer SL, Badesch DB, Barst RJ, Farber HW, Lindner JR, Mathier MA, McGoon MD, Park MH, Rosenson RS, Rubin LJ, Tapson VF, Varga J, American College of Cardiology Foundation Task Force on Expert Consensus Documents. American Heart Association. American College of Chest Physicians. American Thoracic Society, Inc. Pulmonary Hypertension Association. ACCF/AHA 2009 expert consensus

document on pulmonary hypertension a report of the American College of Cardiology Foundation Task Force on Expert Consensus Documents and the American Heart Association developed in collaboration with the American College of Chest Physicians; American Thoracic Society, Inc.; and the Pulmonary Hypertension Association. J Am Coll Cardiol. 2009;53(17): 1573–619.

81. Savarese G, Paolillo S, Costanzo P, D'Amore C, Cecere M, Losco T, et al. Do changes of 6-minute walk distance predict clinical events in patients with pulmonary arterial hypertension? A meta-analysis of 22 randomized trials. J Am Coll Cardiol. 2012;60(13):1192–201.

82. Gomberg-Maitland M, Bull TM, Saggar R, Barst RJ, Elgazayerly A, Fleming TR, et al. New trial designs and potential therapies for pulmonary artery hypertension. J Am Coll Cardiol. 2013;62(25 Suppl):D82–91.

83. Simonneau G, Robbins IM, Beghetti M, Channick RN, Delcroix M, Denton CP, et al. Updated clinical classification of pulmonary hypertension. J Am Coll Cardiol. 2009;54(1 Suppl):S43–54.

84. Simonneau G, Gatzoulis MA, Adatia I, Celermajer D, Denton C, Ghofrani A, et al. Updated clinical classification of pulmonary hypertension. J Am Coll Cardiol. 2013;62(25 Suppl):D34–41.

85. Frost AE, Badesch DB, Barst RJ, Benza RL, Elliott CG, Farber HW, et al. The changing picture of patients with pulmonary arterial hypertension in the United States: how REVEAL differs from historic and non-US Contemporary Registries. Chest. 2011;139(1):128–37.

86. Archer SL, Weir EK, Wilkins MR. Basic science of pulmonary arterial hypertension for clinicians: new concepts and experimental therapies. Circulation. 2010;121(18):2045–66.

87. Duffels MG, Engelfriet PM, Berger RM, van Loon RL, Hoendermis E, Vriend JW, et al. Pulmonary arterial hypertension in congenital heart disease: an epidemiologic perspective from a Dutch registry. Int J Cardiol. 2007;120(2):198–204.

88. Denton CP, Hachulla E. Risk factors associated with pulmonary arterial hypertension in patients with systemic sclerosis and implications for screening. Eur Respir Rev. 2011;20(122):270–6.

89. Lau EM, Manes A, Celermajer DS, Galie N. Early detection of pulmonary vascular disease in pulmonary arterial hypertension: time to move forward. Eur Heart J. 2011;32(20):2489–98.

90. Sitbon O, Lascoux-Combe C, Delfraissy JF, Yeni PG, Raffi F, De Zuttere D, et al. Prevalence of HIV-related pulmonary arterial

hypertension in the current antiretroviral therapy era. Am J Respir Crit Care Med. 2008;177(1):108–13.

91. Machado RD, Eickelberg O, Elliott CG, Geraci MW, Hanaoka M, Loyd JE, et al. Genetics and genomics of pulmonary arterial hypertension. J Am Coll Cardiol. 2009;54(1 Suppl):S32–42.

92. Machado RF, Gladwin MT. Pulmonary hypertension in hemolytic disorders: pulmonary vascular disease: the global perspective. Chest. 2010;137(6 Suppl):30S–8.

93. Parent F, Bachir D, Inamo J, Lionnet F, Driss F, Loko G, et al. A hemodynamic study of pulmonary hypertension in sickle cell disease. N Engl J Med. 2011;365(1):44–53.

94. Fonseca GH, Souza R, Salemi VM, Jardim CV, Gualandro SF. Pulmonary hypertension diagnosed by right heart catheterisation in sickle cell disease. Eur Respir J. 2012;39(1):112–8.

95. Thenappan T, Shah SJ, Rich S, Gomberg-Maitland M. A USA-based registry for pulmonary arterial hypertension: 1982–2006. Eur Respir J. 2007;30(6):1103–10.

96. Ling Y, Johnson MK, Kiely DG, Condliffe R, Elliot CA, Gibbs JS, et al. Changing demographics, epidemiology, and survival of incident pulmonary arterial hypertension: results from the pulmonary hypertension registry of the United Kingdom and Ireland. Am J Respir Crit Care Med. 2012;186(8):790–6.

Chapter 2
Molecular Biological Aspects, Therapeutic Targets and New Treatment Strategies

Dongmin Shao, Laura Price, and Stephen John Wort

Introduction

The term pulmonary arterial hypertension (PAH) describes a rare group of diseases characterized by raised pulmonary vascular resistance, resulting from vascular remodelling in the pre-capillary resistance arterioles (<100 μm in cross-sectional diameter) [1]. Left untreated, patients die from right heart failure, with a mortality approaching most serious cancers. To date, most treatment has been focused on the endothelial cell vascular dysfunction seen in these disorders. As such, pulmonary vasodilators, such as endothelin (ET-1)

D. Shao (✉) • L. Price
Section of Vascular Biology, National Heart and Lung Institute, Imperial College, London, UK
e-mail: d.shao@imperial.ac.uk

S. J. Wort
Section of Vascular Biology, National Heart and Lung Institute, Imperial College, London, UK

Department of Pulmonary Hypertension, Royal Brompton Hospital, Sydney Street, London SW3 6NP, UK
e-mail: s.wort@imperial.ac.uk

B. Madden (ed.), *Treatment of Pulmonary Hypertension*,
Current Cardiovascular Therapy,
DOI 10.1007/978-3-319-13581-6_2,
© Springer International Publishing Switzerland 2015

receptor antagonists, prostacyclin (PGI_2) analogues and phosphodiesterase type V inhibitors (enhancing endogenous nitric oxide (NO)) have improved both morbidity and mortality. Indeed, there is continuing development into new and improved drugs that target these established pathways. Recent examples are the dual ET-1 receptor antagonist, macitentan [2], and the soluble guanylate cyclase activator, riociguat [3]. However, none are a cure and the treated mortality rate is still unacceptable [4]. Further research into the molecular mechanisms underpinning the pathogenesis of PAH has led to the discovery of new putative pathways that may allow the targeting of vascular remodelling itself; such "reverse remodelling" may provide a cure for this devastating disease in the future and remains the "holy grail".

This review will present a molecular biological overview of the pathobiology of PAH, the basis behind current treatments and molecular targets that may provide future therapies.

Definition of Pulmonary Arterial Hypertension

PAH is defined as a mean pulmonary artery pressure (mPAP) of greater than 25 mmHg at rest, with normal left sided filling pressures (left ventricular end diastolic pressure (LVEDP) or pulmonary artery wedge pressure (PAWP) less than 15 mmHg).

Histology of PAH

The characteristic histological finding in all causes of PAH is hyperplasia of vascular cells comprising the three layers of the vascular wall i.e., intima (endothelial cells), media (smooth muscle cells) and adventitia (fibroblasts and resultant connective tissue) (Fig. 2.1). The changes described are thought to originate in the resistance vessels (<100 μm cross sectional diameter), with "secondary" changes occurring in the larger,

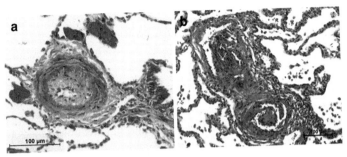

FIGURE 2.1 Histology showing remodelled pulmonary arteries in idiopathic pulmonary arterial hypertension (iPAH). Photographs of paraffin-embedded haematoxylin and eosin-stained human lung sections from patients with iPAH following lung transplantation. Medium sized pulmonary arteries with medial hypertrophy and intimal proliferation (**a**) and plexiform lesions (**b**) (Images kindly supplied by Dr Peter Dorfmuller, Paris)

conduit vessels at a later stage. In severe cases, plexiform lesions, consisting of proliferation of immature endothelial cells and myofibroblasts, are observed, positioned after divisions of the arterial tree and contributing to obstruction of blood flow. *In situ* thrombosis in affected vessels is common and perivascular immune cell infiltrates are seen, suggesting a role for inflammation, either in initiating or propagating the vascular remodelling process. Despite the similarities seen across conditions associated with PAH, there is a more recent realisation that there are distinct histological differences that may be characteristic of the underlying associated condition [5].

Pathogenesis of PAH

It is likely that the pathogenesis of PAH is a multi-hit phenomenon, similar to that described in cancer biology. As such there is evidence for an underlying genetic predisposition and known "hits" such as increased blood flow (Eisenmenger Syndrome), auto-antibodies (connective tissue disease), exposure to drugs (such as appetite suppressants), viruses (HIV) and inflammation. PAH is considered to be a progressive disease, although the exact rate of progression and the exact order of events remain unknown. Most authorities consider that endothelial damage and resulting endothelial dysfunction is the initial hit. This is characterised by an imbalance of vaso-active hormone production and loss of endothelial barrier integrity, leading to exposure of circulating mediators to the underlying smooth muscle. Activated smooth muscle cells may then respond by proliferation and autocrine production of mediators such as ET-1, which may propagate the process.

Endothelial Dysfunction

The following section will describe the abnormalities seen in the vasoactive hormones ET-1, PGI_2 and NO associated with endothelial dysfunction.

ET-1

ET-1 is both a vasoconstrictor and mitogen that is mainly produced by the endothelium. However, under inflammatory conditions, the vascular smooth muscle is another important source. In patients with PAH there is increased production of ET-1 by the endothelium, and to a lesser extent smooth muscle, in remodelled vessels [6]. Furthermore, circulating plasma levels of ET-1 are raised in patients with PAH [7] and, importantly, increased circulating levels of ET-1 correlate with increased right atrial pressure, increased pulmonary vascular resistance, decreased pulmonary artery oxygen saturation and increased mortality [8–11].

NO

NO is a gaseous, lipophilic, free radical produced by the endothelium, which acts, via activation of soluble guanylate cyclase, to increase intra-cellular cyclic GMP. This, in turn, results in vascular smooth muscle relaxation (vasodilation) by altering intracellular Ca^{2+} concentrations. With relevance to vascular remodelling, NO also inhibits leukocyte adhesion, platelet aggregation, thrombus formation, and vascular proliferation [12, 13]. Reduced levels of endothelial nitric oxide synthetase (eNOS) are observed in the lungs of patients with idiopathic PAH [14]. There are several other molecular mechanisms explaining the decreased NO bioavailability in PAH including increased levels of endogenous competitive inhibitor of constitutive eNOS (such as asymmetric dimethylarginine (ADMA)), eNOS "uncoupling", decreased L-Arginine levels and increased NO scavenging by haemoglobin and reactive oxygen species (ROS) [15, 16].

PGI_2

The major active metabolite of arachidonic acid (AA), PGI_2, is a critical endogenous regulator of vascular homeostasis. PGI_2 is produced in vascular endothelial cells and acts on neighbouring vascular smooth muscle, as well as circulating platelets [17]. PGI_2 is an agonist of adenylate cyclase and therefore a potent vasodilator with antithrombotic properties, acting via increase in cyclic AMP [17, 18]. An imbalance in AA metabolism has been demonstrated in patients with idiopathic PAH, with evidence for decreased PGI_2 and increased thromboxane (TXA_2) urinary metabolites [19]. Furthermore, expression of the key enzyme for PGI_2 synthesis PGI_2 synthase (PGIS), is reduced in pulmonary arteries of patients with PAH [20].

In the following sections we will describe the pre-disposing factors and secondary "hits" that may contribute to vascular remodelling.

Genetic Predisposition

Although idiopathic and heritable PAH are rare, an improved understanding of the genetics of heritable PAH (constituting up to 10 % of "idiopathic" PAH cases) has revealed pathobiological mechanisms that may be relevant to PAH associated with other, more common, conditions. Specifically, the genetic defect underlying the majority (80 %) of cases of heritable PAH was identified as heterozygous germ-line mutations in the gene encoding the bone morphogenetic protein receptor (BMPR)-II [21, 22], a member of transforming growth factor-beta (TGF-β) superfamily (Fig. 2.2). Similar mutations have been found in 20 %

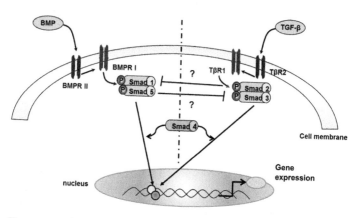

FIGURE 2.2 Schematic representation of bone morphogenetic protein (BMP) signalling via Smads and the interaction with the transforming growth factor (TGF)-β pathway. *Abbreviations: BMP bone morphogenetic protein, BMPR BMP receptor, TGF transforming growth factor, TβR- TGF receptor; Smad- Mothers Against Decapentaplegic Homolog protein.* Bone morphogenetic protein receptors (BMPRs) are members of the transforming growth factor-β (TGF-β) superfamily. Ligand binding to the BMPR I-II complex activates the signalling molecules Smad 1 and 5, which together with the co-Smad 4 regulate gene expression. In particular, it appears that in the healthy cell, most of the action of these Smads is to down-regulate cell proliferation genes and increase pro-apoptotic genes. BMPR II mutations, seen in patients with idiopathic PAH result in disrupted Smad 1, 5 signalling, and a relative increase in pro-proliferative/anti-apoptotic genes. It remains unclear how the BMPR I-II pathway interacts with traditional TGF-β signalling via Smad 2, 3

of sporadic cases of idiopathic PAH [23]. Segregation analysis of affected families demonstrates that the disease is autosomal dominant often with markedly reduced penetrance (as low as 20 %) [24]. Furthermore, it appears that the predominant genetic mechanism is haplo-insufficiency [25]. A reduction in BMPR II expression has now been observed in other, more common, forms of human PAH [26] and in animal models of PAH [27, 28]. Indeed, selective deletion of BMPR II in animal models results in PAH, although usually at levels milder than in human disease [29]. More recently mutations have been found in genes encoding other members of the TGF-beta superfamily, such as endoglin, ALK-1 and SMAD 8 [30–32]. Interestingly, in a few affected families, abnormalites have also been found in non-TGF-beta superfamily molecules such as caveolin-1 [33] and KCNK3 [34].

Blood Flow

Clearly increased flow is a key initiating event (and likely propagating factor) in the pathogenesis of Eisenmenger syndrome (ES), where increased left-to-right blood flow through a congenital shunt leads to perseverance of the fetal type (high pressure) pulmonary circulation. It is also known that turbulent, non-linear, flow leads to increased shear stress and activation of endothelial cells, through NF-κB dependent mechanisms [35–37]. Areas of turbulent flow are associated with formation of atherosclerosis, overlying thrombosis and vessel wall rupture in patients with ES [38].

There are several lines of evidence to suggest that BMPR II dependent signalling may be important in regulating responses to flow. Firstly, one of the ligands for BMPR II, BMP4 is involved in regulating inflammation and subsequent atherosclerosis production in endothelial cells [39, 40]. Endothelial cells release BMP4 in response to oscillatory flow, which in turn enhances monocyte adhesion. Co-release of endogenous inhibitors of BMP4, such as noggin and follicostatin, acts to attenuate this inflammatory pathway [41]. Secondly, BMPR II provides a site for multiple proteins to cluster in the plasma membrane, including cytoskeleton proteins, protein kinases (e.g., LIM kinase, Src, PKC, MAPKs) transcriptional factors (e.g., CtBP, NF κBp50) and transient receptor potential canonical 1 (TRPC1), a non-selective Ca2+ channel, some of which have been described as taking part in flow sensing mechanisms[42–47]. Interestingly, mRNA and protein/activity of TRPs are upregulated in lung and smooth muscle cells isolated from patients with idiopathic PAH (although the BMPR II status was unknown [48]). Thirdly, in the pig model of flow associated systemic-pulmonary shunt induced PH, concomitant to the rise of pulmonary vascular resistance and arteriolar medial thickness, there is a decrease in expression of BMPR II (and its co-receptor BMPR Ia). Conversely, pre-treatment with the angiotensin receptor antagonist, losartan decreased shunt-induced pulmonary vascular resistance and medial thickness with a return to normal of the BMPR II expression [49]. These data would suggest a close correlation of BMPR II function and shear stress response in vascular cells. However, this also raises an important question as to whether patients with BMPR II mutation are genetically more susceptible to aberrations in shear stress patterns generated by disturbed blood flow; BMPR II mutations could result in abnormality of intracellular response to blood flow, e.g., Ca^{2+} influx or intracellular Ca^{2+} release (TRPC1), cytoskeleton rearrangement (LIM kinase), and gene expression (PKC, Src, NF κB, MAPKs) or BMPs.

Drugs and Toxins

PAH is associated with a variety of drugs and toxins [50]. The most common class of drugs implicated is appetite suppressants, which include drugs such as dexfenfluramine. As these drugs are involved in serotonin signalling (see later section), it is likely that serotonin plays an important role in the pathogenesis of PAH associated with these drugs. However, there is an ever increasing list of drugs associated with the development of PAH (see Table 2.1), the latest being interferons [51]. The most well documented toxic insult ("toxic inflammatory PH") occurred after ingestion of adulterated food oil. This led to acute lung injury associated with eosinophilia and myalgia [52]. PAH occurred in 20 % of hospitalized patients, 2–4 months from onset and in 8 % of longer-term survivors.

TABLE 2.1 Classification for drugs and toxins as risk factors for the development of PAH

Classification of risk associated with drug/toxin	Drug/Toxin
Definite group	Aminorex
	Fenfluramine
	Dexfenfluramine
	Toxic rapeseed oil
	Benfluorex
	SSRIs
Likely group	Amphetamines
	L-Tryptophan
	Methamphetamines
	Dasatinib
Possible group	Cocaine
	Phenylpropanolamine
	St. John's wort
	Chemotherapeutic agents
	Interferon α and β
	Amphetamine-like drugs
Unlikely group	Oral contraceptives
	Estrogen
	Cigarette smoking

Adopted from Nice World Congress 2013 guidelines http://www.sciencedirect.com/science/article/pii/S0735109713058725#

Viruses and Parasites

Viruses

The prevalence of PAH in patients infected with HIV is estimated at around 0.5 % [53]. The onset of PAH in these patients confers a worse prognosis [54] . The precise mechanism by which HIV leads to pulmonary vascular remodelling is unknown, but it is likely to be a multifactorial process, and at least in part related to the induction of proinflammatory cytokines and growth factors from the induced chronic state of immune activation. Unsurprisingly, altered BMPR II signaling is likely to be involved [55], although germ-line BMPR II mutations are not usual in these cases [54]. HIV virus has never been detected in vascular lesions [56]; therefore, indirect action by HIV proteins is likely. For example, the envelope protein glycoprotein-120 (responsible for HIV binding and entry into macrophages) has been shown to induce apoptosis and increase ET-1 secretion from endothelial cells *in vitro* [57]. Furthermore, HIV-1 negative factor (*nef*) antigen, crucial for maintenance of the HIV viral load, has been localized to cells within complex vascular lesions in these patients [58], with a proposed mechanism being an increase in endothelial cells apoptosis followed by the emergence of apoptosis-resistant endothelial cells with a hyperproliferative phenotype [59]. Other viruses have also been implicated in the pathogenesis of PAH. For instance, genes coding for human γ herpes virus 8 (or Kaposi sarcoma-associated herpes virus) proteins have been detected in plexiform lesions [60]. In support of this observation, human γ herpes virus 8 infection of pulmonary microvascular endothelial cells *in vitro* results in an apoptosis-resistant cell phenotype [61], as well as a reduction in BMPR II expression [62]. Furthermore, chronic active Epstein-Barr virus infection has been associated with high circulating IL-6 levels in human, and with the development of PAH [63]. However, there is some controversy in these associations and it remains possible that there are geographical differences in possible infectious insults [64–66].

Parasites

Schistosomiasis is likely to be the most common cause of PAH worldwide: 200 million people are infected, and the associated prevalence is 2–5 % [67]. The development of PAH is thought to follow hepatosplenic infection with *Schistosoma mansoni* and the subsequent development of portal hypertension: after entering the skin, the fresh-water parasite migrates to the lungs and then to the portal venous system, where it matures [68]. The deposition of eggs in liver veins leads to presinusoidal granulomatous inflammation, peri-portal fibrosis, and portal hypertension. The resultant opening of portocaval shunts both increases pulmonary blood flow and creates a pathway for eggs to lodge in the pulmonary capillaries [67, 68]. Histologically, pulmonary vascular lesions are similar to those seen in idiopathic PAH, including the presence of plexiform lesions [69]. The development of schistosomiasis-associated PAH is thought to be due to the deposition of eggs in lung tissue causing mechanical vessel impaction and focal arteritis, inflammation relating to the formation of granulomas around the eggs, and increased pulmonary blood flow. The contribution of inflammation to vascular remodelling in this setting is not well understood. However, using murine models, it appears that a switch from a Th1 to a Th2 immune response is important [70, 71]. Although these models are important in enhancing our understanding of this globally important cause of PAH, the phenotype does not accurately reflect human disease in that there is less portopulmonary pulmonary hypertension.

Inflammation

Inflammation is present in all forms of PAH. However, how inflammation may contribute to the pathogenesis of PAH is not clear (Fig. 2.3.). It is possible that inflammation may initiate vascular remodelling ("initial hit"), be integral in its propagation ("secondary hit"), or just be a reactive response to ongoing remodelling ("bystander" phenomenon). Initial

48   D. Shao et al.

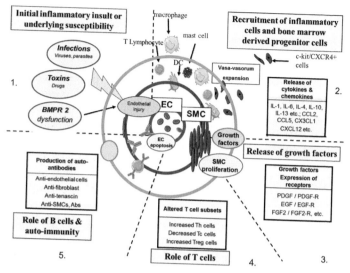

Figure 2.3 The role of inflammation on the pathogenesis of pulmonary arterial hypertension. It is likely that there are 5 stages to the influence of inflammation on pulmonary vascular remodelling: *1* Initial inflammatory insult and/or underlying genetic susceptibility; *2* Recruitment of inflammatory cells and bone marrow derived progenitor cells; *3* Release of inflammatory mediators by either vascular cells themselves or associated inflammatory cells; *4* Role of T cells-it is likely that T cells in some way regulate the inflammatory process; *5* Role of B cells and auto-immunity-there is increasing evidence for anti-bodies against key vascular elements driving the inflammatory process

hits may include infections, drugs, or toxins (see previous sections). There may be a relationship between such an inflammatory hit and other factors such as BMPR II status [72], which may alter the subsequent inflammatory response. Whatever the exact relationship, there is evidence for activation of both the innate immune system (activation of macrophages/monocytes) and adaptive immunity (through specific T-cell and B-cell receptors). The cytokines and chemokines subsequently produced may propagate further inflammatory processes and, either on their own, or together with production of growth factors, drive vascular remodelling processes.

Evidence for Inflammatory Cells

T Cells

T cells are essential components of the adaptive immune response. Several lines of evidence support a role for T cells in the development of PAH. In animal models, the athymic nude rat (without T cells) develops PAH more readily than those with intact T-cell production [73]. In the monocrotaline animal model, depletion of Th cells, as well as those of Th2, ameliorates the extent of PAH, again suggesting the importance of a Th2 antigen-driven immune response [74]. Whereas T-cell infiltrates are increased in patients with idiopathic PAH [75, 76], it appears that there is a decrease in CD8+ cytotoxic (Tc) cells and an increase in regulatory (Treg) cells [77]. The precise role of Treg cells in PAH is currently being investigated.

B Cells

B cells generate antibodies to specific antigenic epitopes. Levels of antinuclear antibodies are increased in patients with PAH [78], and autoantibodies directed against endothelial cells [79] and fibroblasts [80] have been described. These autoantibodies may play a role by inducing adhesion molecule expression [81] or inducing endothelial cell apoptosis [82], which may, in turn, contribute to the apoptosis-resistant phenotype. Finally, the development of PAH in patients with systemic sclerosis is seen in association with specific subsets of human leukocyte antigen alleles [83], although the significance of this remains uncertain.

Mast Cells

Accumulation of mast cells has been described in several types of PAH [84, 85]. A recent study has identified an increase in c-kit-positive cells (including mast cells) in remodelled vessels, as well as mobilization of bone marrow-derived circulating progenitor cells [86]. The increase in mast cell numbers consists mainly of the chymase-secreting subset, numbers of which correlate with the hemodynamic severity of the disease [85]. It is possible that secreted substances from mast cells may be directly vasoactive or have secondary effects such as increased production of matrix metalloproteinases, with consequent involvement in vascular remodelling [84, 87].

Monocytes/Macrophages and Dendritic Cells (DC)

Macrophages are the universal phagocytes that differentiate from tissue monocytes. Along with DC, they are professional antigen-presenting cells, displaying antigen bound to major histocompatibility complex class 2, ready for recognition by T cells. Increased numbers of all these cell types are present around remodelled vessels in PAH [88] . Furthermore, apart from being more numerous in patients with idiopathic PAH, these cells are more "activated" as determined by enhanced nuclear NF-kB immunohistochemical staining [89].

Endothelial Progenitor Cells

Endothelial progenitor cells (EPCs) were first discovered in adult human peripheral blood as a population of CD34 or kinase insert domain receptor (KDR)-positive peripheral blood mononuclear cells which were able to differentiate into mature endothelial cells and were involved in neovascularisation [90]. EPCs are likely to constitute a pool of circulating cells driven from bone marrow in response to stimuli such as tissue ischaemia and vascular damage, and contribute to vascular repair and postnatal neovascularization [91, 92].

Recent animal and clinic studies have suggested that EPCs may be involved in the pathogenesis and progression of PAH [92–94]. For instance, in the mouse hypoxia model of pulmonary hypertension, whole bone marrow transplantation of enhanced green fluorescent protein (GFP)-transgenic mice to lethally irradiated Chimeric mice resulted in the mobilisation of GFP$^+$ cells to remodelling pulmonary arteries [95, 96].

Furthermore, in the lung from patients with PAH, an upregulation of progenitor cell markers such as CD133 and c-Kit in remodelled arteries is observed, especially in plexiform lesions [97]. In these patients, levels of circulating EPCs (CD34$^+$CD133$^+$VEGFR2$^+$) were increased; however, the ability to form vascular networks from late-outgrowth EPCs (CD34$^+$CD146$^+$vWF$^+$CD133$^{+/-}$) was impaired [97].

Evidence for Cytokines/Chemokines

Cytokines

Interleukin (IL)-1-β

IL-1-β is a potent proinflammatory cytokine. In human PAH, serum concentrations are raised [98] and these correlate with a worse outcome [99]. IL-1-β is produced in larger amounts in the monocrotaline animal model, compared with the chronic hypoxic model of pulmonary hypertension [82]. Furthermore, repeated treatment with an IL-1 receptor antagonist reduces pulmonary hypertension and right ventricular hypertrophy in the monocrotaline model, although not in the chronic hypoxia counterpart [100].

IL-6

IL-6 is another proinflammatory cytokine synthesized by many cell types. Plasma concentrations of IL-6 are elevated in idiopathic PAH [98], and they correlate with severity of disease and with increased mortality [99]. In patients with systemic sclerosis, elevated circulating IL-6 concentrations predict the presence of associated PAH [101]. Elevated serum IL-6 concentrations also correlate with hemodynamic severity in pulmonary hypertension associated with COPD [102] and in other forms of PAH, including sickle cell disease-associated PAH [103]. Pulmonary IL-6 production is also increased in experimental pulmonary hypertension and is thought to reflect increased production by both inflammatory cells and vascular cells [104, 105]. In turn, IL-6 has many effects on inflammatory and vascular cells that may promote vascular remodelling. These include accumulation of perivascular T lymphocytes [106], stimulation of endothelial cells to produce chemokines [107], promotion of pulmonary artery smooth muscle cell and endothelial cell proliferation [99,105].

IL-13

IL-13 is a cytokine secreted by many cells, especially Th2 cells and mast cells. It is important in forming granulomata in response to parasites (including schistosomiasis) and its effects on immune cells are similar to those of IL-4. Loss of IL-13 signaling reduces pulmonary vascular remodeling in models of pulmonary hypertension and its effects on T cells suggest an indirect role in regulating Th2 responsiveness [70, 74]. A relative increase in the negative-regulating decoy receptor, IL-13Rα2, is observed in pulmonary arterial smooth muscle cells from patients with idiopathic PAH compared with the active receptors (IL-13Rα1 and IL-4R), as well as in monocrotaline and hypoxic pulmonary hypertension models [108]. Perhaps surprisingly, IL-13 is antiproliferative to pulmonary arterial smooth muscle cells *in vitro*, with an associated reduction in ET-1 release [108]. Overall, these data suggest that dysregulated signalling of this Th2 cytokine is likely to contribute to vascular remodelling in PAH.

Chemokines

Monocyte Chemoattractant Protein(MCP-1)

MCP-1 (or CCL2) is a chemokine produced by vascular cells that stimulates monocytes/macrophage activation and migration, with actions mediated via the chemokine (C-C motif) receptor. Elevated levels of MCP-1 are found in the plasma and lung of patients with idiopathic PAH [109], although they do not correlate with disease severity. Furthermore, vascular smooth muscle cells and endothelial cells from patients with idiopathic PAH release high levels of MCP-1. In addition, vascular smooth muscle cells from patients with idiopathic PAH express increased levels of the chemokine (C-C motif) receptors, exhibit exaggerated migratory and proliferative responses to MCP-1, and these can be blocked by MCP-1 antibodies [109]. Interestingly, an anti-MCP-1 monoclonal antibody has been used in patients with rheumatoid arthritis in a randomized controlled trial, but not yet in PAH [110].

Regulated on Activation, Normal T-cell Expressed and Secreted (RANTES)

RANTES (or CCL5) is a chemokine that mediates the trafficking and homing of T lymphocytes, monocytes, basophils, eosinophils, and natural killer cells through different chemokine receptors [111]. Pulmonary RANTES mRNA is elevated in patients with PAH and shown to be of endothelial cell origin [5, 89, 111]. However, the role of RANTES in the pathogenesis and progression in PAH has not been elucidated.

Fractalkine (CX3CL1)

Fractalkine (CX3CL1) is a chemokine expressed as a soluble or as a membrane-bound form. The effects of fractalkine are mediated through the receptor, CX3CR1, expressed by many cell types. Elevated concentrations of soluble fractalkine are seen in patients with PAH [112], although the association of such elevation with disease severity and prognosis is not currently proven. Increase expression of fractalkine mRNA and protein were detected in pulmonary vascular endothelial cells. Furthermore, it has been shown that the CX3CR1 expression and function were upregulated on both CD4+ and CD8+ T lymphocytes in patient with PAH [89, 112]. It is likely that the concomitant increase of expression in ligands in endothelial cells and receptors on T cells may contribute to the perivascular inflammatory cell influx [113]. Fractalkine and CX3CR1 expression were also shown to be upregulated in pulmonary smooth muscle cells in the monocrotaline rat model of pulmonary hypertension. Finally, fractalkine treatment increased pulmonary arterial smooth muscle cell proliferation *in vitro*, indicating a direct role of fractalkine in vascular remodelling [113].

Platelet Derived Growth Factor (PDGF)

PDGF is secreted as a homodimer of genetically distinct but structurally similar polypeptides (chains A-D) [114]. Additionally, only chain A and chain B can form a functional heterodimer. Increased expression of PDGF-A, PDGF-B and PDGF receptor (R)-α, PDGFR-β mRNA and protein have been found in pulmonary arteries from transplanted PAH patients. Further study demonstrated that PDGF-A and PDGF-B proteins were localised in smooth muscle and endothelial cells, whilst PDGFR-α, PDGFR-β proteins predominated in smooth muscle cells in remodelled pulmonary arteries including plexiform lesions. In addition, intense staining of the ligands and receptors has also been observed in perivascular inflammatory infiltrates [115].

PDGF is a strong mitogen for cells of mesenchymal origin including smooth muscle cells and fibroblasts [114, 115]. Imatinib, a well-established tyrosine kinase inhibitor of the kinase BCR-ABL; the receptor for the stem cell factor, c-KIT; and the PDGFR [116], has been shown to have antiproliferative and pro-apoptotic effects on pulmonary artery smooth muscle cells taken from patients with PAH *in vitro* [115], and has also been shown to reverse pulmonary vascular disease in animal models of PAH [117, 118]. See later section for clinical evidence.

Epidermal Growth Factor (EGF)

EGF promotes chemotaxis, mitogenesis and cytoprotection in epithelial and mesenchymal cells through binding to its receptor (EGFR). The EGFR belongs to the ErbB family of tyrosine kinase receptors [119]. EGF has been shown *in vitro* to increase pulmonary arterial smooth muscle cell proliferation [120]. In the monocrotaline animal model of pulmonary hypertension, the use of serine elastase inhibitors has been shown to reverse pulmonary vascular remodelling. In this study it was suggested that serine elastases, by breaking down extracellular matrix, could lead to the release of EGF and promote vascular remodelling [121].

Vascular Endothelial Growth Factor (VEGF)

VEGF is an endothelial cell specific mitogen and a potent angiogenic mediator. VEGF is produced by a variety of cells and has been implicated in physiological and pathological conditions associated with endothelial cell proliferation [122]. It has been suggested that VEGF is important in attenuating the development of PAH possibly by protecting endothelial cells from injury and apoptosis [123, 124]. Indeed, an overall decrease in pulmonary VEGF expression has been reported, in concert with a dramatic decrease in pulmonary vessel number and a significant increase in vessel wall thickness in the monocrotaline model of pulmonary hypertension [125]. Pulmonary VGEF and VEGF receptor were also down regulated in a rat model of pulmonary hypertension associated with idiopathic pulmonary fibrosis [124]. In contrast, serum VEGF levels are increased in systemic sclerosis patients with PAH [126]. Upregulation of VEGF has also been described in association with plexiform lesions, possibly representing an incomplete attempt at revascularization distal to an arteriolar occlusion [122, 127].

Fibroblast Growth Factor 2 (FGF2)

FGF2 is a member of a large family of heparin-binding growth factors. Increased lung and circulating FGF2 levels have been reported in both experimental and human pulmonary hypertension. Abnormally high levels of FGF2 were found in the blood of 51 % and in the urine of 21 % of patients with idiopathic PAH [128] and in 3 animal models: a lamb model of pulmonary hypertension developed by inserting an aortopulmonary vascular bypass graft [129] and the rat chronic hypoxic and monocrotaline models of pulmonary hypertension[130, 131]. It has been shown that excessive autocrine release of endothelial-derived FGF2 in idiopathic PAH contributes to the acquisition and maintenance of an abnormal endothelial cell phenotype *in vitro* and *in vivo*, enhancing proliferation through constitutive activation of ERK1/2 and decreasing apoptosis by increasing BCL2 and

BCL-xL [132]. Finally, a recent study on apelin knockout mice showed that apelin deficiency led to increased expression of FGF2 and its receptor FGFR1 as a consequence of decreased expression of microRNA (miR)-424 and miR-503, which directly target FGF2 and FGFR1[133].

Serotonin (5-hydroxytryptamine, 5-HT)

Serotonin is an important vasoactive and mitogenic compound that is synthesised by endothelial cells and acts on pulmonary arterial smooth muscle cells [134]. The serotonin transporter (5-HTT) is required for serotonin to elicit its mitogenic effects and transgenic mice overexpressing 5-HTT have been shown to spontaneously develop PH. Serotonin receptors (5-HT$_{2B}$) also appears to play important role in mediated vascular remodelling: mice with restricted expression of 5-HT$_{2B}$ receptors in bone marrow cells exacerbate hypoxia or monocrotaline-induced increases in pulmonary pressure and vascular remodeling, whereas restricted elimination of 5-HT$_{2B}$ receptors on bone marrow cells confers a complete resistance to the development of PH [135]. The role of serotonin system in the pathogenesis of PAH was further supported by the development of PAH in a sub-set of patients taking the anorexigenic drugs aminorex and dexfenfluramine. Both of these drugs are 5-HTT substrates and indirect serotinergic agonists [134]. The overexpression of 5-HTT in pulmonary vascular media may be caused by a polymorphism in the promoter region of the human 5-HTT gene which alters the level of transcription or, alternatively, by BMPR II dysfunction [136–139].

Evidence for Autoantibodies/Autoimmune Phenomenon

Anti-endothelial cell antibodies (AECAs) and anti-fibroblast antibodies (AFAs) have been detected in plasma from patients with idiopathic PAH and with systemic sclerosis-associated PAH (SSc-PAH) [79, 80]. AECAs and AFAs from patients with idiopathic PAH and SSc-PAH showed a distinct reactivity profile; AECAs from patients with idiopathic PAH bound more strongly to a 58 kDa band in dermal microvascular endothelial cells and to a 53 kDa band in lung microvascular endothelial cells. AECAs from patients with limited cutaneous SSc with or without PAH bound to two major bands (75 kDa and 85 kDa) in microvascular endothelial cells [79]. One the other hand, AFAs from these patients predominantly bound to 25-, 40-, and 60-kD protein bands [80]. Further study has identified 16 proteins: vimentin, calumenin, tropomyosin 1, heat shock proteins 27 and 70, glucose-6-phosphate-dehydrogenase, phosphatidylinositol 3-kinase, DAP kinase, and others as the target antigens of AFAs [140]. These proteins are involved in regulation of cytoskeletal function, cell contraction, oxidative stress, cell energy metabolism, and other key cellular pathways. Therefore autoantibodies may play an important role in PAH pathogenesis [140].

Current Treatment of PAH

As mentioned before the current treatment of PAH is based on endothelial dysfunction: hence endothelin receptor antagonists are used to counter increased ET-1 levels; phosphodiesterase type V inhibitors enhance endogenous NO levels; exogenous prostanoids replace deficiencies in PGI_2 production. The evidence for and the use of these drugs is covered in depth in separate chapters. It is also worth noting that to improve safety and efficacy, a number of new drugs targeting these pathways have been tested in clinic trials and will be mentioned here.

Macitentan is a novel dual ET-1 receptor antagonist (ERA) with sustained receptor binding and optimised physiochemical properties, leading to enhanced tissue penetration [141, 142], an improved side-effect profile and limited drug–drug interactions [143, 144]; it also has no significant inhibitory effects on hepatic bile salt transport [145] and therefore has the potential for a favourable liver safety profile [146].

In the recently published SERAPHIN study, macitentan was shown to be superior to placebo in reducing the number of combined mortality and morbidity events in a large group of patients with PAH [2].

Riociguat is a first-in-class drug that augments cGMP biosynthesis (and therefore vasodilation) through direct stimulation of the enzyme, soluble guanylate cyclase (sGC) in an NO-independent fashion, and by sensitization of sGC to low endogenous NO levels [147]. Results from a multi-center, open-label, uncontrolled phase II trial involving 75 patients with PAH ($n = 33$) and chronic thromboembolic pulmonary hypertension ($n = 42$) showed that 12 weeks of oral riociguat given 3 times daily conferred improvements in symptoms, NYHA functional class, exercise capacity, NT-proBNP level, and pulmonary hemodynamics [148]. A decrease in systemic arterial diastolic pressure was the only significant side effect reported, with none associated with symptoms leading to a permanent discontinuation of riociguat [148]. Riociguat is also under investigation in other form of PH such as PH associated with chronic obstructive pulmonary disease, with interstitial lung disease or with left ventricular dysfunction [149–151]. Two large multicentre, randomized, double-blind, placebo-controlled phase III studies have just been published. In PATENT-1, riociguat was shown to be superior to placebo in terms of 6MWT and haemodynamics in patients with PAH [152]. In CHEST-1 riociguat resulted in greater 6MWT and improved haemodynamics in CTEPH patients, either inoperable or with persistent PAH post pulmonary endarterectomy [153].

Future Therapeutic Targets

The following section will cover future potential targets, many of which may target vascular remodelling itself, rather than endothelial cell dysfunction.

PDGF/Tyrosine Kinase Inhibitors

Imatinib, a PDGF/tyrosine kinase receptor inhibitor, was initially shown to be beneficial in a patient with vasodilator-resistant, severe idiopathic PAH [154]. This effect was sustained after 6 months of treatment [154]. A Phase II trial involved 59 patients who were classified as FC II to IV PAH and had an inadequate response to previous therapy were enrolled in a 24 weeks study. The imatinib treated group showed a mean improvement of 22 m in 6MWD compared with a decline of 1 m in the placebo group, although this difference was not significant [155]. However, significant improvements were seen in pulmonary vascular resistance (PVR) (imatinib −300 versus placebo −78 dyn.s.cm-5; $p < 0.01$) and cardiac output (imatinib +0.6 versus placebo −0.1 L/min-1; $p = 0.02$). In the recently published Phase III study, IMPRES, imatinib was used as add-on therapy for advanced patients with PAH who were symptomatic despite treatment with two or more PAH-specific therapies. The imatinib treated group showed significantly improvement in exercise capacity and haemodynamics. However, imatinib did not provide a benefit in terms of FC, time to clinical worsening or mortality [156]. There was also a higher incidence of intracranial haemorrhage in the imatanib treated group. As yet it is not known whether further tyrosine kinase receptor inhibitors will have a better efficacy to side-effect profile. Indeed, dasatinib has been shown to induce PAH in certain patients [157].

The EGF receptor tyrosine kinase inhibitors gefitinib, erlotinib and lapatinib have been tested in rats with monocrotaline-induced pulmonary hypertension. These inhibitors have been shown to inhibit EGF-induced smooth muscle cell proliferation *in vitro* [120]. However, at their highest tolerated dose there was no significant improvement in RV systolic pressure or hypertrophy in animal models. Therefore, more work needed to evaluate the potential of EGFR antagonists as the treatment of PAH.

Epigenetic Modulators

Epigenetics describes changes in phenotype or in gene expression states independent of DNA sequence and include chromatin remodelling, DNA methylation, histone modification and RNA interference. Epigenetic modifications can be inherited or acquired *de novo*, and provide a mechanism that allows the stable propagation of gene activity states from one generation of cells to the next [158]. It has been shown that epigenetic modifications are involved in many diseases mechanisms including cancer, asthma, several hereditary disorders and recently PAH [159, 160].

DNA Methylation

In the heritable fawn hooded rat pulmonary hypertension model, the expression of superoxide dismutase 2 (SOD2) is decreased and yet no mutations are found in the SOD2 gene [161, 162]. However, CpG islands in the SOD2 gene are selectively hypermethylated, which result in ~50 % reduction of SOD2 expression in pulmonary arterial smooth muscle cells from fawn hooded rats compared to those from genetically matched rats [161].

Histone Methylation and Acetylation

It has been shown that constitutive eNOS expression is increased 6-fold in pulmonary vascular endothelial cells derived from a neonatal rodent persistent pulmonary hypertension of the newborn (PPHN) model. The eNOS upregulation was associated with increased H3 and H4 histone acetylation in the eNOS promoter [163] and a small decrease in eNOS methylation. Indeed, increased histone deacetylase (HDAC1 and HDAC5) expression and activity has been found in lungs from patients with idiopathic PAH. Treatment with the HDAC inhibitors, valproic acid, and suberoylanilide hydroxamic acid, reduced the constitutive proliferative phe-notype of adventitial fibroblasts and rhomboidal cells from hypoxic rat *in vitro*, and attenuated the development and ameliorated established pulmonary hypertension in a chronic hypoxic rat model [164].

MicroRNAs (miRNAs)

Micro RNAs are small, non-coding RNA molecules that regu-late gene expression. miRNAs often target groups of genes that are related in terms of function. There is an increasing literature describing associations of miRNAs with the develop-ment of pulmonary hypertension both in *in vivo* models and in human disease [165–167]. For instance miR 150 is downregu-lated in the plasma and lungs of patients with idiopathic PAH, and is associated with poorer outcome [168]. Work is currently underway to develop methods to target miRNAs as a novel therapy for PAH and other cardiovascular diseases [169].

Anti-Inflammatory/Immunosuppressive Treatments

There are reports of successful treatment of patients with PAH associated with lupus and mixed connective tissue disease with immunosuppressive agents [170]. Furthermore, a case study reported successful treatment of a patient with Castleman's-related PAH with the anti-IL-6 monoclonal anti-body, tocilizumab [171]. Interestingly, rapamycin, an immuno-suppressive agent, has also been investigated in animal models of PAH. Rapamycin is also a potent anti-proliferative agent, and has been shown to be effective in preventing the RV wall thickening in rat monocrotaline model [172]. In addition, rapamycin also inhibited the proliferation of pulmonary vas-cular cells *in vitro* and reversed pulmonary vascular remodel-ling in mice hypoxia-induced pulmonary hypertension model [173]. Finally, the steroid dexamethasone, has been shown to reverse the haemodynamic and structural changes seen in the monocrotaline model of pulmonary hypertension and prednisolone inhibits proliferation of pulmonary artery smooth muscle cells from patients with idiopathic PAH *in vitro* [174, 175]. Therefore, anti-inflammatory therapy including immunosuppressants steroids, rapamycin and tocilizumab, may provide novel treatments in the future.

Novel Vasoactive Factors

Apelin

Apelin is a vasodilatory peptide which is thought to play a role in angiogenesis and regulate endothelial and smooth muscle cell apoptosis and proliferation [176]. Interestingly, patients with PAH have lower levels of apelin [176]. Currently, clinical trials are testing whether the administrating apelin is beneficial in humans with PAH.

Vasoactive Intestinal Peptide (VIP)

VIP is also a vasodilator [177]. VIP Knockout mice showed significant increases in right ventricular (RV) systolic pressures, vascular remodelling, and inflammation [178], which was attenuated by treatment with VIP. Two clinic trials showed conflicting results. A multicentre Phase II study in 56 patients with PAH suggested that there was no reduction in PVR, or increase in exercise capacity over 12 weeks compared with placebo [179]. The other, single centre, open-label study of eight patients found that haemodynamics and 6MWD were improved following 3 months' treatment with VIP [180].

Endothelial Nitric Oxide Synthase (eNOS) Couplers

Endothelial nitric oxide synthase can mediate the production of both vasorelaxants and vasoconstrictors: the coupling of eNOS could therefore have a twofold impact on the balance of vasoactive factors released by the endothelial cells [181]. A pilot study of the eNOS coupler, sapropterin dihydrochloride, showed significant improvements in exercise capacity and the treatment was well tolerated, although NO synthesis was not effected [182].

IP Receptor Agonists

The IP receptor is the main receptor for PGI_2. Selexipag, a non-prostanoid, selective IP receptor agonist was recently used in a Phase 2, proof of concept study in patients with PAH. Compared to placebo, there was a significant decrease in PVR with an acceptable side-effect tolerability profile [183]. Given these favourable results a large Phase 3 study (Grython, Actelion Pharmaceuticals) is now underway.

Serotonin Receptor Antagonism

The serotonin receptor antagonist, terguride, has been shown to prevent the development and progression of monocrotaline-induced pulmonary hypertension in rats [184]. However, a 16-week study in 78 patients with PAH showed no overall significant improvements in PVR or other endpoints. Subgroup analysis found that PVR significantly improved in patients who were also treated with an ERA [185].

Rho-kinases

The small GTPase, RhoA and its downstream effectors, ROCK1 and ROCK2, regulate many essential cellular processes such as cell contraction, migration, proliferation, survival, and differentiation. There was a twofold increase in Rho kinase and RhoA activity in lungs from patients with idiopathic PAH as compared to control patients [186].

The activity of ROCK was closely related to the disease duration. In addition, beneficial effects of fasudil [187] and SB-772077-B [188] specific ROCK inhibitors, has been observed in different animal models of pulmonary hypertension [189–193]. However, ROCK inhibitors appear to have serious systemic side effects. Hence, inhalation form of fasudil has been trialed in 15 PAH patients[193] and in 19 patients with high-altitude pulmonary hypertension [194]. This treatment was shown to significantly reduce mPAP and decrease PVR.

Peroxisome Proliferator-Activated Receptor-γ (PPARγ)

PPARγ is a transcription factor which is also a downstream target of BMPR2 signalling. On formation of a complex with catenin, PPARγ triggers the transcription of several genes that appear to be associated with PAH, such as apelin [195] and apoE [196]. Endothelial or smooth muscle cell specific PPARγ knockout mice have been shown to develop pulmonary hypertension [196, 197]. Treatment of rats with experimental pulmonary hypertension using the PPARγ agonist rosiglitazone attenuated the development of hypoxia-induced pulmonary hypertension [198]. Interestingly, PPARγ antagonists pioglitazone and rosiglitazone have been shown to be potent vasodilator on isolated human pulmonary arteries [199].

Cell Therapy

Administration of EPCs in rats with monocrotaline-induced pulmonary hypertension led to the prevention of pulmonary hypertension and restoration of pulmonary microvasculature structure [200]. Pulmonary hypertension and Cell Therapy (PHACeT) is a clinical trial ongoing in Canada in order to assess safety of administrating autologous mononuclear cells transduced with eNOS in patients with isiopathic PAH [201].

Associated to this safety study, efficacy of EPC infusion have been reported in adult and children patients with idiopathic PAH with improvement on exercise capacity and pulmonary hemodynamics [202, 203].

Summary

This chapter has described the molecular biological aspects that underpin both current and future treatment of patients with PAH. It has emphasized the shift away from treating the abnormalities associated with endothelial dysfunction, towards therapy aimed at reversing pulmonary vascular remodelling. Only then will we be able to make a significant impact on the morbidity and mortality associated with this devastating condition.

References

1. Galie N, et al. Guidelines for the diagnosis and treatment of pulmonary hypertension. Eur Respir J. 2009;34(6):1219–63.
2. Pulido T, et al. Macitentan and morbidity and mortality in pulmonary arterial hypertension. N Engl J Med. 2013;369(9):809–18.
3. Bonderman D, et al. Riociguat for patients with pulmonary hypertension caused by systolic left ventricular dysfunction: a phase IIb double-blind, randomized, placebo-controlled, dose-ranging hemodynamic study. Circulation. 2013;128(5):502–11.
4. Humbert M, et al. Survival in patients with idiopathic, familial, and anorexigen-associated pulmonary arterial hypertension in the modern management era. Circulation. 2010;122(2):156–63.
5. Dorfmuller P, et al. Inflammation in pulmonary arterial hypertension. Eur Respir J. 2003;22(2):358–63.
6. Giaid A, et al. Expression of endothelin-1 in the lungs of patients with pulmonary hypertension. N Engl J Med. 1993;328(24): 1732–9.
7. Stewart DJ, et al. Increased plasma endothelin-1 in the early hours of acute myocardial infarction. J Am Coll Cardiol. 1991;18(1):38–43.

8. Cacoub P, et al. Endothelin-1 in pulmonary hypertension. N Engl J Med. 1993;329(26):1967–8.

9. Galie N, et al. Role of pharmacologic tests in the treatment of primary pulmonary hypertension. Am J Cardiol. 1995;75(3):55A–62.

10. Cacoub P, et al. Endothelin-1 in the lungs of patients with pulmonary hypertension. Cardiovasc Res. 1997;33(1):196–200.

11. Nootens M, et al. Neurohormonal activation in patients with right ventricular failure from pulmonary hypertension: relation to hemodynamic variables and endothelin levels. J Am Coll Cardiol. 1995;26(7):1581–5.

12. Mayer B, Hemmens B. Biosynthesis and action of nitric oxide in mammalian cells. Trends Biochem Sci. 1997;22(12):477–81.

13. Lincoln TM, et al. Nitric oxide–cyclic GMP pathway regulates vascular smooth muscle cell phenotypic modulation: implications in vascular diseases. Acta Physiol Scand. 1998;164(4):507–15.

14. Giaid A, Saleh D. Reduced expression of endothelial nitric oxide synthase in the lungs of patients with pulmonary hypertension. N Engl J Med. 1995;333(4):214–21.

15. Zuckerbraun BS, George P, Gladwin MT. Nitrite in pulmonary arterial hypertension: therapeutic avenues in the setting of dysregulated arginine/nitric oxide synthase signalling. Cardiovasc Res. 2011;89(3):542–52.

16. Steinhorn RH. Nitric oxide and beyond: new insights and therapies for pulmonary hypertension. J Perinatol. 2008;28 Suppl 3:S67–71.

17. Vane J, Corin RE. Prostacyclin: a vascular mediator. Eur J Vasc Endovasc Surg. 2003;26(6):571–8.

18. Gryglewski RJ, et al. Arterial walls are protected against deposition of platelet thrombi by a substance (prostaglandin X) which they make from prostaglandin endoperoxides. Prostaglandins. 1976;12(5):685–713.

19. Christman BW, et al. An imbalance between the excretion of thromboxane and prostacyclin metabolites in pulmonary hypertension. N Engl J Med. 1992;327(2):70–5.

20. Tuder RM, et al. Prostacyclin synthase expression is decreased in lungs from patients with severe pulmonary hypertension. Am J Respir Crit Care Med. 1999;159(6):1925–32.

21. Lane KB, et al. Heterozygous germline mutations in BMPR2, encoding a TGF-beta receptor, cause familial primary pulmonary hypertension. Nat Genet. 2000;26(1):81–4.

22. Deng Z, et al. Familial primary pulmonary hypertension (gene PPH1) is caused by mutations in the bone morphogenetic protein receptor-II gene. Am J Hum Genet. 2000;67(3):737–44.

23. Thomson JR, et al. Sporadic primary pulmonary hypertension is associated with germline mutations of the gene encoding BMPR-II, a receptor member of the TGF-beta family. J Med Genet. 2000;37(10):741–5.

24. Loyd JE, Primm RK, Newman JH. Familial primary pulmonary hypertension: clinical patterns. Am Rev Respir Dis. 1984; 129(1):194–7.

25. Machado RD, et al. BMPR2 haploinsufficiency as the inherited molecular mechanism for primary pulmonary hypertension. Am J Hum Genet. 2001;68(1):92–102.

26. Atkinson C, et al. Primary pulmonary hypertension is associated with reduced pulmonary vascular expression of type II bone morphogenetic protein receptor. Circulation. 2002;105(14):1672–8.

27. Rondelet B, et al. Signaling molecules in overcirculation-induced pulmonary hypertension in piglets: effects of sildenafil therapy. Circulation. 2004;110(15):2220–5.

28. Takahashi H, et al. Downregulation of type II bone morphogenetic protein receptor in hypoxic pulmonary hypertension. Am J Physiol Lung Cell Mol Physiol. 2006;290(3):L450–8.

29. Hong KH, et al. Genetic ablation of the BMPR2 gene in pulmonary endothelium is sufficient to predispose to pulmonary arterial hypertension. Circulation. 2008;118(7):722–30.

30. Brenner L, Chung WK. Clinical and molecular genetic features of hereditary pulmonary arterial hypertension. Comp Physiol. 2011;1(4):1721–8.

31. Chida A, et al. Missense mutations of the BMPR1B (ALK6) gene in childhood idiopathic pulmonary arterial hypertension. Circ J. 2012;76(6):1501–8.

32. Shintani M, et al. A new nonsense mutation of SMAD8 associated with pulmonary arterial hypertension. J Med Genet. 2009;46(5):331–7.

33. Austin ED, et al. Whole exome sequencing to identify a novel gene (caveolin-1) associated with human pulmonary arterial hypertension. Circ Cardiovasc Genet. 2012;5(3):336–43.

34. Ma L, et al. A novel channelopathy in pulmonary arterial hypertension. N Engl J Med. 2013;369(4):351–61.

35. Partridge J, et al. Laminar shear stress acts as a switch to regulate divergent functions of NF-kappaB in endothelial cells. FASEB J. 2007;21(13):3553–61.

36. Silver AE, Vita JA. Shear-stress-mediated arterial remodeling in atherosclerosis: too much of a good thing? Circulation. 2006;113(24):2787–9.

37. Davis ME, et al. Shear stress regulates endothelial nitric-oxide synthase promoter activity through nuclear factor kappaB binding. J Biol Chem. 2004;279(1):163–8.

38. Broberg CS, et al. Pulmonary arterial thrombosis in eisenmenger syndrome is associated with biventricular dysfunction and decreased pulmonary flow velocity. J Am Coll Cardiol. 2007;50(7):634–42.

39. Sorescu GP, et al. Bone morphogenic protein 4 produced in endothelial cells by oscillatory shear stress induces monocyte adhesion by stimulating reactive oxygen species production from a nox1-based NADPH oxidase. Circ Res. 2004; 95(8):773–9.

40. Sorescu GP, et al. Bone morphogenic protein 4 produced in endothelial cells by oscillatory shear stress stimulates an inflammatory response. J Biol Chem. 2003;278(33):31128–35.

41. Chang K, et al. Bone morphogenic protein antagonists are coexpressed with bone morphogenic protein 4 in endothelial cells exposed to unstable flow in vitro in mouse aortas and in human coronary arteries: role of bone morphogenic protein antagonists in inflammation and atherosclerosis. Circulation. 2007; 116(11):1258–66.

42. Lehoux S, Castier Y, Tedgui A. Molecular mechanisms of the vascular responses to haemodynamic forces. J Intern Med. 2006;259(4):381–92.

43. Ando J, Yamamoto K. Vascular mechanobiology: endothelial cell responses to fluid shear stress. Circ J. 2009;73(11):1983–92.

44. Hassel S, et al. Proteins associated with type II bone morphogenetic protein receptor (BMPR-II) and identified by two-dimensional gel electrophoresis and mass spectrometry. Proteomics. 2004;4(5):1346–58.

45. Wong WK, Knowles JA, Morse JH. Bone morphogenetic protein receptor type II C-terminus interacts with c-Src: implication for a role in pulmonary arterial hypertension. Am J Respir Cell Mol Biol. 2005;33(5):438–46.

46. Perron JC, Dodd J. ActRIIA and BMPRII Type II BMP receptor subunits selectively required for Smad4-independent BMP7-evoked chemotaxis. PLoS One. 2009;4(12), e8198.

47. Sharif-Naeini R, et al. TRP channels and mechanosensory transduction: insights into the arterial myogenic response. Pflugers Arch. 2008;456(3):529–40.

48. Yu Y, et al. Enhanced expression of transient receptor potential channels in idiopathic pulmonary arterial hypertension. Proc Natl Acad Sci U S A. 2004;101(38):13861–6.

49. Rondelet B, et al. Prevention of pulmonary vascular remodeling and of decreased BMPR-2 expression by losartan therapy in shunt-induced pulmonary hypertension. Am J Physiol Heart Circ Physiol. 2005;289(6):H2319–24.

50. Price LC, et al. Inflammation in pulmonary arterial hypertension. Chest. 2012;141(1):210–21.

51. George PM, et al. Evidence for the involvement of type I interferon in pulmonary arterial hypertension. Circ Res. 2014;114(4): 677–88.

52. James TN. The toxic oil syndrome. Clin Cardiol. 1994;17(9):463–70.

53. Barnier A, et al. Improvement of HIV-related pulmonary hypertension after the introduction of an antiretroviral therapy. Eur Respir J. 2009;34(1):277–8.

54. Nunes H, et al. Prognostic factors for survival in human immunodeficiency virus-associated pulmonary arterial hypertension. Am J Respir Crit Care Med. 2003;167(10):1433–9.

55. Caldwell RL, et al. HIV-1 TAT represses transcription of the bone morphogenic protein receptor-2 in U937 monocytic cells. J Leukoc Biol. 2006;79(1):192–201.

56. Mette SA, et al. Primary pulmonary hypertension in association with human immunodeficiency virus infection. A possible viral etiology for some forms of hypertensive pulmonary arteriopathy. Am Rev Respir Dis. 1992;145(5):1196–200.

57. Kanmogne GD, Primeaux C, Grammas P. Induction of apoptosis and endothelin-1 secretion in primary human lung endothelial cells by HIV-1 gp120 proteins. Biochem Biophys Res Commun. 2005;333(4):1107–15.

58. Marecki JC, et al. HIV-1 Nef is associated with complex pulmonary vascular lesions in SHIV-nef-infected macaques. Am J Respir Crit Care Med. 2006;174(4):437–45.

59. Voelkel NF, Cool CD, Flores S. From viral infection to pulmonary arterial hypertension: a role for viral proteins? AIDS. 2008;22 Suppl 3:S49–53.

60. Cool CD, et al. Expression of human herpesvirus 8 in primary pulmonary hypertension. N Engl J Med. 2003;349(12): 1113–22.

61. Bull TM, et al. Human herpesvirus-8 infection of primary pulmonary microvascular endothelial cells. Am J Respir Cell Mol Biol. 2008;39(6):706–16.

62. Durrington HJ, et al. Identification of a lysosomal pathway regulating degradation of the bone morphogenetic protein receptor type II. J Biol Chem. 2010;285(48):37641–9.
63. Hashimoto T, et al. Pulmonary arterial hypertension associated with chronic active Epstein-Barr virus infection. Intern Med. 2011;50(2):119–24.
64. Valmary S, et al. Human gamma-herpesviruses Epstein-Barr virus and human herpesvirus-8 are not detected in the lungs of patients with severe pulmonary arterial hypertension. Chest. 2011;139(6):1310–6.
65. Bendayan D, et al. Absence of human herpesvirus 8 DNA sequences in lung biopsies from Israeli patients with pulmonary arterial hypertension. Respiration. 2008;75(2):155–7.
66. Henke-Gendo C, et al. Absence of Kaposi's sarcoma-associated herpesvirus in patients with pulmonary arterial hypertension. Am J Respir Crit Care Med. 2005;172(12):1581–5.
67. Graham BB, et al. Schistosomiasis-associated pulmonary hypertension: pulmonary vascular disease: the global perspective. Chest. 2010;137(6 Suppl):20S–9.
68. Lapa M, et al. Cardiopulmonary manifestations of hepatosplenic schistosomiasis. Circulation. 2009;119(11):1518–23.
69. Tuder RM. Pathology of pulmonary arterial hypertension. Semin Respir Crit Care Med. 2009;30(4):376–85.
70. Graham BB, et al. Schistosomiasis-induced experimental pulmonary hypertension: role of interleukin-13 signaling. Am J Pathol. 2010;177(3):1549–61.
71. Crosby A, et al. Pulmonary vascular remodeling correlates with lung eggs and cytokines in murine schistosomiasis. Am J Respir Crit Care Med. 2010;181(3):279–88.
72. Song Y, et al. Inflammation, endothelial injury, and persistent pulmonary hypertension in heterozygous BMPR2-mutant mice. Am J Physiol Heart Circ Physiol. 2008;295(2):H677–90.
73. Cool CD, et al. Pathogenesis and evolution of plexiform lesions in pulmonary hypertension associated with scleroderma and human immunodeficiency virus infection. Hum Pathol. 1997;28(4):434–42.
74. Daley E, et al. Pulmonary arterial remodeling induced by a Th2 immune response. J Exp Med. 2008;205(2):361–72.
75. Tuder RM, et al. Exuberant endothelial cell growth and elements of inflammation are present in plexiform lesions of pulmonary hypertension. Am J Pathol. 1994;144(2):275–85.

76. Perros F, et al. Pulmonary lymphoid neogenesis in idiopathic pulmonary arterial hypertension. Am J Respir Crit Care Med. 2012;185(3):311–21.
77. Ulrich S, et al. Increased regulatory and decreased CD8+ cytotoxic T cells in the blood of patients with idiopathic pulmonary arterial hypertension. Respiration. 2008;75(3): 272–80.
78. Rich S, et al. Antinuclear antibodies in primary pulmonary hypertension. J Am Coll Cardiol. 1986;8(6):1307–11.
79. Tamby MC, et al. Anti-endothelial cell antibodies in idiopathic and systemic sclerosis associated pulmonary arterial hypertension. Thorax. 2005;60(9):765–72.
80. Tamby MC, et al. Antibodies to fibroblasts in idiopathic and scleroderma-associated pulmonary hypertension. Eur Respir J. 2006;28(4):799–807.
81. Carvalho D, et al. IgG antiendothelial cell autoantibodies from scleroderma patients induce leukocyte adhesion to human vascular endothelial cells in vitro. Induction of adhesion molecule expression and involvement of endothelium-derived cytokines. J Clin Invest. 1996;97(1):111–9.
82. Bordron A, et al. The binding of some human antiendothelial cell antibodies induces endothelial cell apoptosis. J Clin Invest. 1998;101(10):2029–35.
83. Gladman DD, et al. HLA markers for susceptibility and expression in scleroderma. J Rheumatol. 2005;32(8):1481–7.
84. Heath D, Yacoub M. Lung mast cells in plexogenic pulmonary arteriopathy. J Clin Pathol. 1991;44(12):1003–6.
85. Hamada H, et al. Increased expression of mast cell chymase in the lungs of patients with congenital heart disease associated with early pulmonary vascular disease. Am J Respir Crit Care Med. 1999;160(4):1303–8.
86. Montani D, et al. C-kit-positive cells accumulate in remodeled vessels of idiopathic pulmonary arterial hypertension. Am J Respir Crit Care Med. 2011;184(1):116–23.
87. Vajner L, et al. Acute and chronic hypoxia as well as 7-day recovery from chronic hypoxia affects the distribution of pulmonary mast cells and their MMP-13 expression in rats. Int J Exp Pathol. 2006;87(5):383–91.
88. Perros F, et al. Dendritic cell recruitment in lesions of human and experimental pulmonary hypertension. Eur Respir J. 2007; 29(3):462–8.

89. Price LC, et al. Nuclear factor kappa-B is activated in the pulmonary vessels of patients with end-stage idiopathic pulmonary arterial hypertension. PLoS One. 2013;8(10), e75415.

90. Ward MR, Stewart DJ, Kutryk MJ. Endothelial progenitor cell therapy for the treatment of coronary disease, acute MI, and pulmonary arterial hypertension: current perspectives. Catheter Cardiovasc Interv. 2007;70(7):983–98.

91. Yang JX, et al. Endothelial progenitor cell-based therapy for pulmonary arterial hypertension. Cell Transplant. 2013;22(8):1325–36.

92. Diller GP, et al. Circulating endothelial progenitor cells in patients with Eisenmenger syndrome and idiopathic pulmonary arterial hypertension. Circulation. 2008;117(23):3020–30.

93. Anjum F, et al. Characterization of altered patterns of endothelial progenitor cells in sickle cell disease related pulmonary arterial hypertension. Pulm Circ. 2012;2(1):54–60.

94. Junhui Z, et al. Reduced number and activity of circulating endothelial progenitor cells in patients with idiopathic pulmonary arterial hypertension. Respir Med. 2008;102(7):1073–9.

95. Marsboom G, et al. Sustained endothelial progenitor cell dysfunction after chronic hypoxia-induced pulmonary hypertension. Stem Cells. 2008;26(4):1017–26.

96. Davie NJ, et al. Hypoxia-induced pulmonary artery adventitial remodeling and neovascularization: contribution of progenitor cells. Am J Physiol Lung Cell Mol Physiol. 2004;286(4):L668–78.

97. Toshner M, et al. Evidence of dysfunction of endothelial progenitors in pulmonary arterial hypertension. Am J Respir Crit Care Med. 2009;180(8):780–7.

98. Humbert M, et al. Increased interleukin-1 and interleukin-6 serum concentrations in severe primary pulmonary hypertension. Am J Respir Crit Care Med. 1995;151(5):1628–31.

99. Soon E, et al. Elevated levels of inflammatory cytokines predict survival in idiopathic and familial pulmonary arterial hypertension. Circulation. 2010;122(9):920–7.

100. Voelkel NF, et al. Interleukin-1 receptor antagonist treatment reduces pulmonary hypertension generated in rats by monocrotaline. Am J Respir Cell Mol Biol. 1994;11(6):664–75.

101. Gourh P, et al. Plasma cytokine profiles in systemic sclerosis: associations with autoantibody subsets and clinical manifestations. Arthritis Res Ther. 2009;11(5):R147.

102. Eddahibi S, et al. Interleukin-6 gene polymorphism confers susceptibility to pulmonary hypertension in chronic obstructive pulmonary disease. Proc Am Thorac Soc. 2006;3(6):475–6.

103. Niu X, et al. Angiogenic and inflammatory markers of cardio-pulmonary changes in children and adolescents with sickle cell disease. PLoS One. 2009;4(11), e7956.
104. Miyata M, et al. Pulmonary hypertension in rats. 2. Role of interleukin-6. Int Arch Allergy Immunol. 1995;108(3):287–91.
105. Savale L, et al. Impact of interleukin-6 on hypoxia-induced pulmonary hypertension and lung inflammation in mice. Respir Res. 2009;10:6.
106. Steiner MK, et al. Interleukin-6 overexpression induces pulmonary hypertension. Circ Res. 2009;104(2):236–44, 28p following 244.
107. Imaizumi T, Yoshida H, Satoh K. Regulation of CX3CL1/frac-talkine expression in endothelial cells. J Atheroscler Thromb. 2004;11(1):15–21.
108. Hecker M, et al. Dysregulation of the IL-13 receptor system: a novel pathomechanism in pulmonary arterial hypertension. Am J Respir Crit Care Med. 2010;182(6):805–18.
109. Sanchez O, et al. Role of endothelium-derived CC chemokine ligand 2 in idiopathic pulmonary arterial hypertension. Am J Respir Crit Care Med. 2007;176(10):1041–7.
110. Brennan F, Beech J. Update on cytokines in rheumatoid arthri-tis. Curr Opin Rheumatol. 2007;19(3):296–301.
111. Dorfmuller P, et al. Chemokine RANTES in severe pul-monary arterial hypertension. Am J Respir Crit Care Med. 2002;165(4):534–9.
112. Balabanian K, et al. CX(3)C chemokine fractalkine in pul-monary arterial hypertension. Am J Respir Crit Care Med. 2002;165(10):1419–25.
113. Perros F, et al. Fractalkine-induced smooth muscle cell prolifera-tion in pulmonary hypertension. Eur Respir J. 2007;29(5):937–43.
114. Heldin CH. Structural and functional studies on platelet-derived growth factor. EMBO J. 1992;11(12):4251–9.
115. Perros F, et al. Platelet-derived growth factor expression and function in idiopathic pulmonary arterial hypertension. Am J Respir Crit Care Med. 2008;178(1):81–8.
116. Grimminger F, Schermuly RT. PDGF receptor and its antagonists: role in treatment of PAH. Adv Exp Med Biol. 2010;661:435–46.
117. Ciuclan L, et al. Imatinib attenuates hypoxia-induced pul-monary arterial hypertension pathology via reduction in 5-hydroxytryptamine through inhibition of tryptophan hydroxylase 1 expression. Am J Respir Crit Care Med. 2013;187(1):78–89.

118. Tu L, et al. A critical role for p130Cas in the progression of pulmonary hypertension in humans and rodents. Am J Respir Crit Care Med. 2012;186(7):666–76.
119. Dreux AC, et al. The epidermal growth factor receptors and their family of ligands: their putative role in atherogenesis. Atherosclerosis. 2006;186(1):38–53.
120. Dahal BK, et al. Role of epidermal growth factor inhibition in experimental pulmonary hypertension. Am J Respir Crit Care Med. 2010;181(2):158–67.
121. Ye CL, Rabinovitch M. Inhibition of elastolysis by SC-37698 reduces development and progression of monocrotaline pulmonary hypertension. Am J Physiol. 1991;261(4 Pt 2):H1255–67.
122. Tuder RM, et al. Expression of angiogenesis-related molecules in plexiform lesions in severe pulmonary hypertension: evidence for a process of disordered angiogenesis. J Pathol. 2001;195(3):367–74.
123. Sakao S, et al. VEGF-R blockade causes endothelial cell apoptosis, expansion of surviving CD34+ precursor cells and trans-differentiation to smooth muscle-like and neuronal-like cells. FASEB J. 2007;21(13):3640–52.
124. Farkas L, et al. VEGF ameliorates pulmonary hypertension through inhibition of endothelial apoptosis in experimental lung fibrosis in rats. J Clin Invest. 2009;119(5):1298–311.
125. Partovian C, et al. Heart and lung VEGF mRNA expression in rats with monocrotaline- or hypoxia-induced pulmonary hypertension. Am J Physiol. 1998;275(6 Pt 2):H1948–56.
126. Papaioannou AI, et al. Serum VEGF levels are related to the presence of pulmonary arterial hypertension in systemic sclerosis. BMC Pulm Med. 2009;9:18.
127. Jonigk D, et al. Plexiform lesions in pulmonary arterial hypertension composition, architecture, and microenvironment. Am J Pathol. 2011;179(1):167–79.
128. Benisty JI, et al. Elevated basic fibroblast growth factor levels in patients with pulmonary arterial hypertension. Chest. 2004;126(4):1255–61.
129. Wedgwood S, et al. Fibroblast growth factor-2 expression is altered in lambs with increased pulmonary blood flow and pulmonary hypertension. Pediatr Res. 2007;61(1):32–6.
130. Chen W, Yan H. Change of level of basic fibroblast growth factor in serum of rats with chronic hypoxic pulmonary hypertension. Hua Xi Yi Ke Da Xue Xue Bao. 1998;29(4):372–5.

131. Arcot SS, et al. Basic fibroblast growth factor alterations during development of monocrotaline-induced pulmonary hypertension in rats. Growth Factors. 1995;12(2):121–30.
132. Tu L, et al. Autocrine fibroblast growth factor-2 signaling contributes to altered endothelial phenotype in pulmonary hypertension. Am J Respir Cell Mol Biol. 2011;45(2):311–22.
133. Kim J, et al. An endothelial apelin-FGF link mediated by miR-424 and miR-503 is disrupted in pulmonary arterial hypertension. Nat Med. 2013;19(1):74–82.
134. Adnot S, et al. Serotonin transporter and serotonin receptors. Handb Exp Pharmacol. 2013;218:365–80.
135. Launay JM, et al. Serotonin 5-HT2B receptors are required for bone-marrow contribution to pulmonary arterial hypertension. Blood. 2012;119(7):1772–80.
136. Zhang H, et al. Association between serotonin transporter (SERT) gene polymorphism and idiopathic pulmonary arterial hypertension: a meta-analysis and review of the literature. Metabolism. 2013;62(12):1867–75.
137. Ulasli SS, et al. Associations between endothelial nitric oxide synthase A/B, angiotensin converting enzyme I/D and serotonin transporter L/S gene polymorphisms with pulmonary hypertension in COPD patients. Mol Biol Rep. 2013;40(10):5625–33.
138. Thomas M, et al. Targeting the serotonin pathway for the treatment of pulmonary arterial hypertension. Pharmacol Ther. 2013;138(3):409–17.
139. Baloira A, et al. Polymorphisms in the serotonin transporter protein (SERT) gene in patients with pulmonary arterial hypertension. Arch Bronconeumol. 2012;48(3):77–80.
140. Terrier B, et al. Identification of target antigens of antifibroblast antibodies in pulmonary arterial hypertension. Am J Respir Crit Care Med. 2008;177(10):1128–34.
141. Gatfield J, et al. Slow receptor dissociation kinetics differentiate macitentan from other endothelin receptor antagonists in pulmonary arterial smooth muscle cells. PLoS One. 2012;7(10), e47662.
142. Iglarz M, et al. Pharmacology of macitentan, an orally active tissue-targeting dual endothelin receptor antagonist. J Pharmacol Exp Ther. 2008;327(3):736–45.
143. Bruderer S, et al. Effect of cyclosporine and rifampin on the pharmacokinetics of macitentan, a tissue-targeting dual endothelin receptor antagonist. AAPS J. 2012;14(1):68–78.

144. Atsmon J, et al. Investigation of the effects of ketoconazole on the pharmacokinetics of macitentan, a novel dual endothelin receptor antagonist, in healthy subjects. Clin Pharmacokinet. 2013;52(8):685–92.

145. Bolli MH, et al. The discovery of N-[5-(4-bromophenyl)-6-[2-[(5-bromo-2-pyrimidinyl)oxy]ethoxy]-4-pyrimidinyl]-N'-propylsulfamide (Macitentan), an orally active, potent dual endothelin receptor antagonist. J Med Chem. 2012;55(17):7849–61.

146. Raja SG. Macitentan, a tissue-targeting endothelin receptor antagonist for the potential oral treatment of pulmonary arterial hypertension and idiopathic pulmonary fibrosis. Curr Opin Investig Drugs. 2010;11(9):1066–73.

147. Ghofrani HA, Grimminger F. Soluble guanylate cyclase stimulation: an emerging option in pulmonary hypertension therapy. Eur Respir Rev. 2009;18(111):35–41.

148. Ghofrani HA, et al. Riociguat for chronic thromboembolic pulmonary hypertension and pulmonary arterial hypertension: a phase II study. Eur Respir J. 2010;36(4):792–9.

149. Hoeper MM, et al. Riociguat for interstitial lung disease and pulmonary hypertension: a pilot trial. Eur Respir J. 2013;41(4):853–60.

150. Schermuly RT, et al. Riociguat for the treatment of pulmonary hypertension. Expert Opin Investig Drugs. 2011;20(4):567–76.

151. Ghio S, et al. Left ventricular systolic dysfunction associated with pulmonary hypertension riociguat trial (LEPHT): rationale and design. Eur J Heart Fail. 2012;14(8):946–53.

152. Ghofrani HA, et al. Riociguat for the treatment of pulmonary arterial hypertension. N Engl J Med. 2013;369(4):330–40.

153. Ghofrani HA, et al. Riociguat for the treatment of chronic thromboembolic pulmonary hypertension. N Engl J Med. 2013;369(4):319–29.

154. Ghofrani HA, Seeger W, Grimminger F. Imatinib for the treatment of pulmonary arterial hypertension. N Engl J Med. 2005;353(13):1412–3.

155. Ghofrani HA, et al. Imatinib in pulmonary arterial hypertension patients with inadequate response to established therapy. Am J Respir Crit Care Med. 2010;182(9):1171–7.

156. Hoeper MM, et al. Imatinib mesylate as add-on therapy for pulmonary arterial hypertension: results of the randomized IMPRES study. Circulation. 2013;127(10):1128–38.

157. Montani D, et al. Pulmonary arterial hypertension in patients treated by dasatinib. Circulation. 2012;125(17):2128–37.

158. Kim GH, et al. Epigenetic mechanisms of pulmonary hypertension. Pulm Circ. 2011;1(3):347–56.
159. Xu XF, Du LZ. Epigenetics in neonatal diseases. Chin Med J (Engl). 2010;123(20):2948–54.
160. Huang JB, et al. Epigenetics: novel mechanism of pulmonary hypertension. Lung. 2013;191(6):601–10.
161. Archer SL, et al. Epigenetic attenuation of mitochondrial superoxide dismutase 2 in pulmonary arterial hypertension: a basis for excessive cell proliferation and a new therapeutic target. Circulation. 2010;121(24):2661–71.
162. Bonnet S, et al. An abnormal mitochondrial-hypoxia inducible factor-1alpha-Kv channel pathway disrupts oxygen sensing and triggers pulmonary arterial hypertension in fawn hooded rats: similarities to human pulmonary arterial hypertension. Circulation. 2006;113(22):2630–41.
163. Xu XF, et al. Epigenetic regulation of the endothelial nitric oxide synthase gene in persistent pulmonary hypertension of the newborn rat. J Hypertens. 2010;28(11):2227–35.
164. Zhao L, et al. Histone deacetylation inhibition in pulmonary hypertension: therapeutic potential of valproic acid and suberoylanilide hydroxamic acid. Circulation. 2012;126(4):455–67.
165. Schlosser K, White RJ, Stewart DJ. miR-26a Linked to Pulmonary Hypertension by Global Assessment of Circulating Extracellular MicroRNAs. Am J Respir Crit Care Med. 2013;188(12):1472–5.
166. Caruso P, et al. A role for miR-145 in pulmonary arterial hypertension: evidence from mouse models and patient samples. Circ Res. 2012;111(3):290–300.
167. Courboulin A, et al. Role for miR-204 in human pulmonary arterial hypertension. J Exp Med. 2011;208(3):535–48.
168. Rhodes CJ, et al. Reduced microRNA-150 is associated with poor survival in pulmonary arterial hypertension. Am J Respir Crit Care Med. 2013;187(3):294–302.
169. Brock M, et al. AntagomiR directed against miR-20a restores functional BMPR2 signalling and prevents vascular remodelling in hypoxia-induced pulmonary hypertension. Eur Heart J. 2014;35(45):3203–11.
170. Meloche J, et al. Anti-inflammatory and immunosuppressive agents in PAH. Handb Exp Pharmacol. 2013;218:437–76.
171. Furuya Y, Satoh T, Kuwana M. Interleukin-6 as a potential therapeutic target for pulmonary arterial hypertension. Int J Rheumatol. 2010;2010:720305.

172. Houssaini A, et al. Rapamycin reverses pulmonary artery smooth muscle cell proliferation in pulmonary hypertension. Am J Respir Cell Mol Biol. 2013;48(5):568–77.
173. Paddenberg R, et al. Rapamycin attenuates hypoxia-induced pulmonary vascular remodeling and right ventricular hypertrophy in mice. Respir Res. 2007;8:15.
174. Ogawa A, et al. Prednisolone ameliorates idiopathic pulmonary arterial hypertension. Am J Respir Crit Care Med. 2011;183(1):139–40.
175. Price LC, et al. Dexamethasone reverses monocrotaline-induced pulmonary arterial hypertension in rats. Eur Respir J. 2010;37:813–22.
176. Andersen CU, et al. Apelin and pulmonary hypertension. Pulm Circ. 2011;1(3):334–46.
177. Hamidi SA, et al. VIP and endothelin receptor antagonist: an effective combination against experimental pulmonary arterial hypertension. Respir Res. 2011;12:141.
178. Stenmark KR, et al. Animal models of pulmonary arterial hypertension: the hope for etiological discovery and pharmacological cure. Am J Physiol Lung Cell Mol Physiol. 2009;297(6):L1013–32.
179. Said SI. Vasoactive intestinal peptide in pulmonary arterial hypertension. Am J Respir Crit Care Med. 2012;185(7):786; author reply 786.
180. Petkov V, et al. Vasoactive intestinal peptide as a new drug for treatment of primary pulmonary hypertension. J Clin Invest. 2003;111(9):1339–46.
181. Kar S, Kavdia M. Modeling of biopterin-dependent pathways of eNOS for nitric oxide and superoxide production. Free Radic Biol Med. 2011;51(7):1411–27.
182. Robbins IM, et al. Safety of sapropterin dihydrochloride (6r-bh4) in patients with pulmonary hypertension. Exp Lung Res. 2011;37(1):26–34.
183. Simonneau G, et al. Selexipag: an oral, selective prostacyclin receptor agonist for the treatment of pulmonary arterial hypertension. Eur Respir J. 2012;40(4):874–80.
184. Dumitrascu R, et al. Terguride ameliorates monocrotaline-induced pulmonary hypertension in rats. Eur Respir J. 2011;37(5):1104–18.
185. Ghofrani HA, et al. Proof-of-concept study to investigate the efficacy, hemodynamics and tolerability of terguride Vs. Placebo in subjects with pulmonary arterial hypertension: results of a double blind, randomised, prospective phase IIa study. Am J Respir Crit Care Med. 2012;185:A2495.

186. Do e Z, et al. Evidence for Rho-kinase activation in patients with pulmonary arterial hypertension. Circ J. 2009;73(9):1731–9.
187. Pankey EA, et al. The Rho kinase inhibitor azaindole-1 has long-acting vasodilator activity in the pulmonary vascular bed of the intact chest rat. Can J Physiol Pharmacol. 2012;90(7):825–35.
188. Dhaliwal JS, et al. Analysis of pulmonary vasodilator responses to SB-772077-B [4-(7-((3-amino-1-pyrrolidinyl)carbonyl)-1-ethyl-1H-imidazo(4,5-c)pyridin-2-yl)-1,2,5-oxadiazol-3-amine], a novel aminofurazan-based Rho kinase inhibitor. J Pharmacol Exp Ther. 2009;330(1):334–41.
189. Abe K, et al. Long-term treatment with a Rho-kinase inhibitor improves monocrotaline-induced fatal pulmonary hypertension in rats. Circ Res. 2004;94(3):385–93.
190. Tawara S, Fukumoto Y, Shimokawa H. Effects of combined therapy with a Rho-kinase inhibitor and prostacyclin on monocrotaline-induced pulmonary hypertension in rats. J Cardiovasc Pharmacol. 2007;50(2):195–200.
191. Nagaoka T, et al. Inhaled Rho kinase inhibitors are potent and selective vasodilators in rat pulmonary hypertension. Am J Respir Crit Care Med. 2005;171(5):494–9.
192. Mouchaers KT, et al. Fasudil reduces monocrotaline-induced pulmonary arterial hypertension: comparison with bosentan and sildenafil. Eur Respir J. 2010;36(4):800–7.
193. Fujita H, et al. Acute vasodilator effects of inhaled fasudil, a specific Rho-kinase inhibitor, in patients with pulmonary arterial hypertension. Heart Vessels. 2010;25(2):144–9.
194. Kojonazarov B, et al. Effects of fasudil in patients with high-altitude pulmonary hypertension. Eur Respir J. 2012;39(2):496–8.
195. Alastalo TP, et al. Disruption of PPARgamma/beta-catenin-mediated regulation of apelin impairs BMP-induced mouse and human pulmonary arterial EC survival. J Clin Invest. 2011;121(9):3735–46.
196. Hansmann G, et al. An antiproliferative BMP-2/PPARgamma/apoE axis in human and murine SMCs and its role in pulmonary hypertension. J Clin Invest. 2008;118(5):1846–57.
197. Guignabert C, et al. Tie2-mediated loss of peroxisome proliferator-activated receptor-gamma in mice causes PDGF receptor-beta-dependent pulmonary arterial muscularization. Am J Physiol Lung Cell Mol Physiol. 2009;297(6):L1082–90.
198. Kim EK, et al. Rosiglitazone attenuates hypoxia-induced pulmonary arterial hypertension in rats. Respirology. 2010;15(4):659–68.

199. Kozlowska H, et al. Relaxation of human pulmonary arteries by PPARgamma agonists. Naunyn Schmiedebergs Arch Pharmacol. 2013;386(5):445–53.
200. Zhao YD, et al. Rescue of monocrotaline-induced pulmonary arterial hypertension using bone marrow-derived endothelial-like progenitor cells: efficacy of combined cell and eNOS gene therapy in established disease. Circ Res. 2005;96(4):442–50.
201. NIH., U. ClinicalTrials.gov. Pulmonary hypertension: assessment of cell therapy (PHACeT) [online], 2010.
202. Wang XX, et al. Transplantation of autologous endothelial progenitor cells may be beneficial in patients with idiopathic pulmonary arterial hypertension: a pilot randomized controlled trial. J Am Coll Cardiol. 2007;49(14):1566–71.
203. Zhu JH, et al. Safety and efficacy of autologous endothelial progenitor cells transplantation in children with idiopathic pulmonary arterial hypertension: open-label pilot study. Pediatr Transplant. 2008;12(6):650–5.

Chapter 3
Current Treatment Strategies, Guidelines and New Therapies

Adam Loveridge, Jenny Bacon, and Brendan Madden

Historically, primary pulmonary hypertension (as it was then termed) has been considered a rapidly progressive, fatal condition with no effective therapies with an average life expectancy of less than 3 years at diagnosis [1]. It has been labelled as a "desperate disease" and upon diagnosis one enters "the kingdom of the near-dead" [2].

In the 1980s, the vasodilatation caused by high dose calcium channel blockers was discovered to have a beneficial effect. These results were shown to improve pulmonary artery pressure, pulmonary vascular resistance, right ventricular hypertrophy and survival. It did however become quickly apparent that the treated population could be clearly sub-divided into two categories – those who responded and those who did not [3].

A. Loveridge • J. Bacon
Cardiothoracic Unit, St. George's Hospital, London, UK
e-mail: jb901@doctors.org.uk; adam.loveridge@stgeorges.nhs.uk

B. Madden (✉)
Division of Cardiac and Vascular Science, St. George's Hospital, London, UK
e-mail: brendan.madden@stgeorges.nhs.uk

B. Madden (ed.), *Treatment of Pulmonary Hypertension*, Current Cardiovascular Therapy, DOI 10.1007/978-3-319-13581-6_3, © Springer International Publishing Switzerland 2015

Over the past 15 years there has been rapid progress in the field, predominantly in the treatment of class 1, pulmonary arterial hypertension (PAH). Several classes of advanced, targeted vasodilator medication have been developed and there is now a wealth of evidence supporting their use. Given the rapid progress being made, optimal treatment strategies are constantly evolving. The three major classes of therapy (namely endothelin receptor antagonists, phosphodiesterase-5 inhibitors and prostacyclin analogues) and the evidence behind their use are discussed below.

Since 2001, all decisions regarding the commencement of targeted vasodilator therapy in the UK and Ireland are made by the National Pulmonary Hypertension Service. There are nine centres as designated by the National Commissioning Group. These are Western Infirmary (Glasgow), Mater Misericordiae University Hospital (Dublin), Freeman Hospital (Newcastle), Royal Hallamshire Hospital (Sheffield), Papworth Hospital (Cambridge) and in London, the Royal Brompton Hospital, Hammersmith Hospital, Royal Free Hospital and Great Ormond Street Hospital [4].

Individual agents have shown both clinical (symptomatic, functional and delayed time to worsening) and haemodynamic improvements and when the trials are taken together there is a survival benefit. A mortality reduction of 43 % was shown by a 2009 meta-analysis of targeted vasodilator therapy versus placebo [5]. Pulmonary arterial hypertension patients can now expect a median prognosis of approximately 9 years at diagnosis, threefold that of the pre-vasodilator era [6] (Fig. 3.1).

Endothelin Receptor Antagonists

Endothelin-1 is a peptide produced by the endothelium with potent vasoconstricting and smooth muscle proliferating properties. It is found at higher concentrations in pulmonary hypertension and has also been implicated in the pathogenesis of atherosclerosis and systemic hypertension. Oral endothelin receptor antagonism has been used since the late 1990s in pulmonary arterial hypertension.

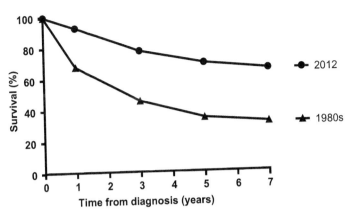

FIGURE 3.1 Survival plot before and after the advent of targeted vasodilator therapy, using REVEAL registry data (2012) of idiopathic and familial PAH matched to that from National Institutes of Health registry (1980s) (Adapted from Benza et al. *Chest* [6] with permission)

The two receptor isoforms A and B are more prominent in pulmonary artery smooth muscle and vascular endothelium respectively. Bosentan and macitentan act on both receptors whereas ambrisentan (and sitaxentan) are selective for endothelin receptor A. Despite endothelin receptor B having vasodilatory effects and playing a role in endothelin-1 clearance, the selective antagonists have not been shown to be clinically superior to date.

Transaminitis is the most important side-effect and hence monthly blood test monitoring is required. Sitaxentan was initially reported to be efficacious and to have a low incidence of hepatic complications [7] but was taken off the market in 2010 due to several reported deaths from hepatotoxicity [8].

Other side-effects of these agents are peripheral oedema, nausea, hypotension, teratogenicity, anaemia, headaches/jaw pain and flushing. Ambrisentan needs to be used with caution in idiopathic pulmonary fibrosis [9].

Bosentan

The BREATHE-1 trial was a 2002 randomised controlled trial (RCT) with 213 idiopathic and associated PAH patients who were highly symptomatic, namely functional class (FC) III or IV. After 16 weeks' treatment, the mean 6 min walk test (6MWT) increased by 35 m and 54 m (125 mg and 250 mg BD respectively versus placebo), and 34–38 % had improved to WHO FC II. In addition the time to clinical worsening was prolonged. There was a 7 % reported transaminitis rate at the higher dose [10].

The EARLY study from Italy in 2008 recruited 185 FC II, group 1 patients. After 6 months, the haemodynamics and symptoms improved and time to clinical worsening was delayed. Pulmonary vascular resistance (PVR) was 83 % of baseline in the treated arm and 6MWT 19 m further between the two arms [11].

Ambrisentan

ARIES 1 and 2 were concurrent double-blind trials involving a total of 394 idiopathic and associated PAH patients who were targeted vasodilator treatment naive and had a 6MWT between 150 and 450 m. The randomisation was to different dosing regimens (2.5, 5 and 10 mg OD) and placebo controlled. The primary end-point of 6MWT increased by between 31 and 54 m with dose dependency seen. Also seen was statistically significant improvement in functional class, health related questionnaire, time to clinical worsening, Borg dyspnoea and BNP level. The initial study time period was 12 weeks but an extension studies showed persistent benefits to 48 weeks and 2 years. Elevation in transaminases was quoted at 3.9 %. Hence ambrisentan is considered to have a safer liver side-effect profile than bosentan [12, 13].

ARIES 3 was an open label, uncontrolled study that broadened the patient selection criteria to include Dana Point groups 3 and 4. Overall 6MWT increased by 21 m. This improvement was seen in groups 1 and 4 but not group

3. The COPD and ILD sub-group demonstrated a slight deterioration in their exercise capacity but their BNP levels did decrease in keeping with the other aetiologies [14].

Macitentan

This novel unselective endothelin receptor antagonist is believed to be more potent due to prolonged binding time and tissue penetration. Macitentan had initially shown promising results in animal models and now has a large international RCT with morbidity benefit supporting its use.

The SERAPHIN study of 742 group 1 patients, with the primary outcome measure of morbidity events and mortality, was reported in 2013 [15]. The study population were mainly FC II and III and approximately 60 % were already taking targeted vasodilator medication, predominantly a phosphodiesterase-5 inhibitor. There was a highly significant reduction in adverse events, usually clinical worsening of PH, and the hazard ration for the 10 mg dose of macitentan compared with placebo was 0.55. There was also a non-significant trend towards mortality benefit. 6MWT and FC also showed significant improvement (the former by 22 m) with a degree of dose dependency. The transaminitis incidence was lower than placebo at 3.5 %.

Phosphodiesterase-5 Inhibitors

Sildenafil, tadalafil and vardenafil are selective cyclic GMP phosphodiesterase type 5 inhibitors which are administered orally. cGMP acts as a second messenger in the nitric oxide pathway and PDE5 is upregulated in the pulmonary hypertension vascular bed. The PDE5 inhibitors prevent the breakdown of cGMP and hence cause potentiation of the endothelial smooth muscle relaxtion of NO. In addition they are believed to be anti-proliferative and have shown pulmonary vascular remodelling in vitro.

Side-effects include postural hypotension (hence the contraindication with concurrent nitrates), visual disturbance including cyanopsia (with cGMP PDE5 particularly prevalent in the retina), headache, hearing loss, flushing and dyspepsia. They are the most recently developed class, with sildenafil first licensed in 2005. Two newer PDE5 inhibitors, tadalafil and vardenafil, are longer acting (hence requiring less frequent administration) and appear to be equally efficacious. Vardenafil may be more potent due to prolonged binding time.

Sildenafil

Case reports, small non-randomised studies and one RCT from the early 2000s first showed the benefit of sildenafil [16–20] but the strongest evidence for its use as monotherapy comes from the SUPER-1 trial. 278 PAH patients were recruited into a 12 week double blind RCT with four arms, placebo versus 20, 40 and 80 mg TDS. The population studied were IPAH, connective tissue disease and a few congential patients post-surgical correction. There was improvement in 6MWT (improved by 45–50 m, which represented 13.0–14.7 %), mean PA pressure (small absolute reduction but statistically significant) and WHO FC (improved by at least one in 7 % of placebo and up to 42 % at the highest dosage) [21]. The same trial population also undertook health related quality of life questionnaires SF-36 and EQ-5D with significant improvement [22].

259 of the above patients underwent a 3 year open label, uncontrolled extension in SUPER-2. Approximately half at least maintained their 6MWT and functional class over the 3 years from pre-treatment baseline. 3 years survival was 79 %. The majority were uptitrated to 80 mg TDS (with good safety profile) and 18 % had had a second agent added by the end [23].

Tadalafil

The PHIRST RCT involved 405 idiopathic or associated PAH patients. The highest dose 40 mg OD increased 6MWT by a mean 44 m after 16 weeks as single agent [24].

Vardenafil

Vardenafil was studied by RCT in treatment naive PAH over 12 weeks in the EVALUATION trial. 6MWT improved by 69 m. Haemodynamics were also significantly improved in terms of pulmonary artery pressure (down 5.3 mmHg), cardiac output (up by 0.39 l/min) and pulmonary vascular resistance (down by 4.7 WU). WHO FC and Borg dyspnoea were also improved. For the first time a PDE5 inhibitor was shown to reduce clinical worsening events, namely death or hospitalisation [25].

Prostacyclin Analogues

Prostacyclin (or prostaglandin I2) is a prostinoid produced by vascular endothelium that has vasodilatory, anti-thrombotic, anti-proliferative and anti-inflammatory properties. The pathway has a significant role in the pathogenesis of pulmonary hypertension. Intravenous epoprostenol was the first advance targeted vasodilator licensed for treatment of PH (in 1998). Several analogues have been developed but the mode of administration remains problematic.

Epoprostenol

Initial trials from the 1990s showed benefit from continuous IV epoprostenol infusion in idiopathic pulmonary arterial hypertension [26–29].

As with the other classes, the best level of evidence comes from group 1 PAH patients who have advanced disease, i.e. WHO FC III or IV. The above unblinded RCT by Barst et al. in 1996 involved 81 such patients and showed statistically significant improvement in terms of exercise tolerance (6MWT differential of 47 m between the arms and functional class improved in 40 % compared with only 3 % in the placebo arm), haemodynamics (PVR reduced by

21 % compared with a 9 % increase in placebo) and even a survival benefit (zero deaths compared with 8) over a 12 week period.

Epoprostenol has a half-life of only a few minutes and consequently does require continuous infusion without interuption. The syringe needs to be changed every 8 h due to the medication degrading unrefrigerated. Specific complications include pump disruption, infusion pain, line thrombosis and infection. Should there be any disruption to the flow then there is a 10–15 min window to rectify matters. If this is unsuccessful then there is the potential for a rebound pulmonary hypertensive crisis and death. Other complications include hypotension, jaw pain, flushing, wheeze, nausea, diarrhoea, agitation and arthralgias.

Treprostinil

Treprostinil is an epoprostenol analogue which has been developed to have greater stability at room temperature. Consequently it has the advantage that is can be given subcutaneously as well as intravenously. Subcutaneously it has been shown to have a survival benefit and improved functional class in PAH patients [30]. Oral preparations are being developed but their efficacy has not been proven to date [31].

Iloprost

Inhaled or nebulised iloprost has been shown to be beneficial in a range of aetiologies including group 1 and group 4 with FC III and IV. It has to be administered every 2–4 h and proves a significant time burden on those using it [32]. There is only limited evidence with the use of intravenous iloprost with its efficacy called into question.

Beraprost

Beraprost as an oral preparation that demonstrates an improvement in symptoms which is only temporary. It appears to work for the first 3–6 months but this is not sustained at the 12 months mark [33, 34].

Selexipag

This novel prostacyclin receptor agonist can be administered orally and has phase 2 evidence behind it. It is discussed later in the novel/future therapies section (Table 3.1).

Combination Therapy

In the future it seems likely that dual or even triple therapy will be commenced at an earlier stage. Randomised controlled trials are being reported every year but have had mixed results to date. All of the following studies are exclusively in group 1 PAH patients.

One relatively early prospective cohort showed the benefit of sildenafil added into iloprost in the context of clinical deterioration [35].

Bosentan and prostanoids in combination in idiopathic PAH has shown contradictory results with the following studies being positive and negative respectively [36, 37]. However the best calibre of evidence comes from the 2006 STEP-1 trial with 67 PAH patients randomised to placebo versus iloprost added into bosentan monotherapy. The 6MWT improvement at 12 weeks was 26 m and 34 % improved functional class (compared with 6 % in placebo arm) [38].

BREATHE 2 saw bosentan added into epoprostenol and although there was a trend towards functional improvement with both therapies, it was not significant [39].

TABLE 3.1 Summary of advanced, targeted pulmonary vasodilator medication

Endothelin receptor antagonists

Side-effects	Hepatic dysfunction, peripheral oedema, nausea, hypotension, teratogenicity, anaemia, headaches/jaw pain and flushing					
Name	Brand name	Route of administration	Initial Dose	Up-titration dose	Monitoring	Notes
Bosentan	Tracleer	Oral	62.5 mg BD	250 mg BD	Monthly liver function required	Interaction with warfarin (bosentan)
Ambrisentan	Volibris	Oral	5 mg OD	10 mg OD		Contra-indicated with cyclosporin
Macitentan	Opsumit	Oral	3 mg OD	10 mg OD		

Phosphodiesterase-5 inhibitors

Side-effects	Postural hypotension, visual disturbance including cyanopsia, headache, hearing loss, flushing and dyspepsia					
Name	Brand name	Route of administration	Initial Dose	Up-titration dose	Monitoring	Notes
Sildenafil	Revatio, Viagra	Oral	20 mg TDS or 25 mg TDS	50 mg TDS	History of visual impairment	Contra-indicated with nitrates
Tadalafil	Adcirca	Oral	20 mg OD	40 mg OD		First line in hepatic dysfunction
Vardenafil	Levitra	Oral	5 mg BD	20 mg BD		

Prostacyclin analogues

Side-effects Hypotension, jaw pain, flushing, wheeze, nausea, diarrhoea, agitation and arthralgias.
Administration may be complicated by pump disruption, infusion pain, line thrombosis and infection

Name	Brand name	Route of administration	Initial Dose	Up-titration dose	Monitoring	Notes
Epoprostenol	Veletri, Flolan	Intravenous	2 ng/kg/min	200 ng/kg/min		High risk of rebound pulmonary hypertension if infusion is disrupted
Treprostinil	Remodulin, Tyvaso	Intravenous, subcutaneous or nebulised	1.25 ng/kg/ min IV/SC	40 ng/kg/min IV/ SC		
Iloprost	Ventavis	Nebulised	2.5 µg 6–9× per day	5 µg 6–9× per day		

Sildenafil plus epoprotenol in 267 class III patients showed significant improvement in a range of clinical and haemodynamic parameters [40].

The PHIRST trial increased 6MWT by 23 m when tadalafil was added into bosentan [24].

The positive SERAPHIN study into macitentan had almost two thirds of its participants already taking a phosphodiesterase-5 inhibitor and revealed a significant morbidity benefit [15].

TRIMUPH in 2010 involved 235 severe patients (functional class III and IV) where inhaled treprostinil was added into bosentan or sildenafil. There was an improvement in the primary end-point of 6 min walk testing (improved by 20 m) but no change in time to clinical worsening or level of dyspnoea [41].

The FREEDOM-C and FREEDOM-C2 trials have been published in the last 12 months. Oral treporostinol, at different dosages, was added to patients already on advanced vasodilators, be that a PDE-5 inhibitor, endothelin receptor antagonist or both. There was no improvement in the primary end-point of 6MWT and there was a 22 % discontinuation rate with high incidence of side-effects. There was however some benefit in secondary outcomes such as dyspnoea [31, 42].

The AMBITION study is evaluating combination ambrisentan and tadalafil versus single agent arms in 614 treatment naive PAH patients and should be publishing in the near future.

Initial triple therapy was evaluated in 10 idiopathic and heritable PAH patients with FC III and IV and haemodynamic severity (cardiac index less than 2 l/min/m^2 or pulmonary vascular resistance more than 12.5 Wood units) at diagnosis. The results were very impressive with all patients at 4 months (n of 7) improving to FC II but one requiring transplantation due to lack of improvement. There was a mean improvement in 6MWT of 164 m, mean PA pressure reduction of 13 mmHg, PVR reduction of 16.7 Wood units and cardiac index improvement of 2.l/min/m^2 which was maintained at (median) 18 months and well tolerated [43].

Calcium Channel Blockers

Prior to the advent of targeted vasodilators, inhaled nitric oxide response was used as a predictor of response to high dose calcium channel blockers. Those not responding had, in addition to the lack of clinical efficacy, a far higher incidence of side-effects including severe complications such as cardiogenic shock and hypoxaemia (due to loss of hypoxic pulmonary vasoconstriction and subsequent worsening V/Q matching).

Vasoreactivity testing (with inhaled nitric oxide or intravenous adenosine/epoprostenol at the time of right heart catheterisation – RHC) should be performed in all group 1 PH patients. Calcium channel blockers are not used as the testing agent due to the high risk of serious side-effects in the non-responders [44]. Testing is relatively contraindicated in pulmonary veno-occlusive disease due to the risk of pulmonary oedema.

The test is considered positive should the mean PA pressure fall by at least 10 mmHg to a value of under 40 mmHg without any fall in the cardiac output. There is approximately a 10 % chance that this will be the case. This rises significantly in the anorexigen induced PH population. The importance of a positive vasoreactivity test is a significantly better prognosis and it is a strong predictor for good response to calcium channel antagonists. High dose, sustained release preparations of nifedipine and diltiazem (with the strongest evidence base) are most commonly used. Observational studies have shown a symptomatic and survival benefit that can be prolonged over years [3].

There is however the suggestion that responders have less severe disease at baseline with a longer duration of symptoms [45]. Consequently they are likely to represent a distinct, more indolent phenotype and there is evidence to show the survival benefit is seen even when not treated with calcium channel blockers [46].

Close follow-up is suggested to ensure the calcium channel antagonist response is maintained (some guidelines suggesting a repeat RHC at 3–4 months) with only 54 % reported to maintain the beneficial response [45]. Targeted vasodilators should be commenced early when the response is not maintained.

Guidelines

The joint European Society of Cardiology (ESC) and European Respiratory Society (ERS) guidelines were published in 2009 [47]. The World Symposium on Pulmonary Hypertension took place in Nice in February/March 2013. Consequently there have been a number of recently published updates to the classification and treatment regimen [48]. The guidelines are summarised below.

A holistic approach to treatment is suggested including general measures (such as oxygen, diuretics and warfarin, as detailed in general measures), exercise, infection prevention, pregnancy advice, psychosocial support, multi-disciplinary approach and palliative care when appropriate.

There are a number of established treatment goals with an evidence basis behind them. Essentially it orientates around keeping patients in the "stable and satisfactory" group and the prevention or reversal of poor prognostic indicators. The precise therapeutic goals are as follows:

- Clinical – no signs of right ventricular failure or history of syncope, WHO functional class I or II, 6MWT >500 m, peak VO_2 >15 ml/min/kg and normal or near-normal BNP;
- Echocardiography – no pericardial effusion and TAPSE >2.0 cm;
- Right heart catheterisation – right atrial pressure <8 mmHg and cardiac index ≥2.5 l/min/m².

First line in the treatment algorithm of PAH patients is the vasoreactivity testing and commencement of calcium channel blockers if positive. In non-responders, choice of targeted vasodilator depends on functional class, with treatment usually indicated when in FC II and above. First line choice is not usually specified due to lack of data. Therefore that choice is made by the treating physician with the knowledge of the individual circumstances to guide therapy for example hepatic or renal dysfunction.

However there are some caveats. The one exception to specified therapy is intravenous epoprostenol as first line in

FC IV. This is also the only group where combination therapy should be considered from the outset. In FC II an endothelin receptor antagonist or phosphodiesterase-5 inhibitor should be considered first line.

Although not always specified in the guidelines, it would be usual practice to routinely uptitrate the dose of single vasodilator if tolerated. Should there be insufficient clinical improvement then this would trigger the addition of initially a second agent and then full triple therapy. Inadequate response is defined as "stable and not satisfactory" (i.e. therapeutic goals not met) or "unstable and deteriorating" (such as the development of right heart failure) in FC II or III. At the most severe end of the spectrum, there is also emphasis on rapidly leaving FC IV.

The precise treatment algorithm with grades of supporting evidence is reproduced below (Fig. 3.2).

There are also guidelines from the American College of Cardiology Foundation and American Heart Association published in 2009 [49]. These are similar to the ESC/ERS guidelines except instead of using functional class to guide treatment, patients are divided into lower and high risk. As per FC IV, high risk patients are suggested to commence intravenous prostanoids but either epoprostenol or treprostinil is suggested. The risk stratification is determined by clinical criteria. High risk criteria being FC IV, rapid progression, right ventricular failure, 6MWT <300 m, peak VO2 <10.4 ml/kg/min, pericardial effusion, significant right ventricular enlargement or dysfunction, right atrial enlargement, RA pressure >20 mmHg, CI <2.0 l/min/m^2 and significantly elevated BNP.

General Measures

Anticoagulation

Several observational, predominantly retrospective, studies performed in the 1980s showed an improvement in survival when taking warfarin in idiopathic pulmonary hypertension. Subgroup analysis from the 1992 calcium channel antagonist

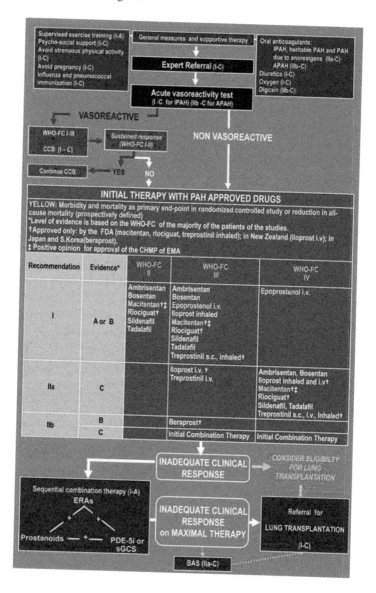

study revealed a 3 year survival benefit from 31 to 62 % with warfarin in the non-responder population [3], albeit those selected out for treatment by non-uniformity on a perfusion scan. A 2006 literature review found a survival benefit in 5 out of 7 studies involving idiopathic PAH [50].

The rationale behind anticoagulation is prothrombotic tendency (with abnormal clotting cascade, platelet function and fibrinolysis) and altered right sided haemodynamics (sluggish flow in dilated atrium and ventricle). Thrombotic arteriopathy has a strong histopathological association with pulmonary arterial hypertension although the cause/effect relationship is unknown [51].

Current best practice is to commence warfarin, in the absence of contraindication, in certain group 1 (namely idiopathic, hereditable and anorexigen induced) and naturally group 4 Dana Point pulmonary hypertension. It is not usually recommended in connective tissue disease associated PH due to an increased bleeding risk. The optimal target INR or functional class for treatment has not been established.

There is currently no data (even in CTEPH) regarding the use of the novel oral anticoagulant agents (such as the direct

FIGURE 3.2 Evidence-based treatment algorithm for pulmonary arterial hypertension patients (for group 1 patients only) (Reproduced from Galiè et al., *Journal of the American College of Cardiology* [48] with permission) Key: *APAH* associated pulmonary arterial hypertension, *BAS* balloon atrial septostomy, *CCB* calcium channel blockers, *ERA* endothelin receptor antagonist, *sGCS* soluble guanylate cyclase stimulators, *IPAH* idiopathic pulmonary arterial hypertension, *i.v.* intravenous, *PDE-5i* phosphodiesterase type-5 inhibitor, *s.c.* subcutaneous, *WHO-FC* World Health Organization functional class

thrombin inhibitor dabigatran and the factor Xa inhibitors rivaroxaban and apixaban) and there are also interactions with endothelin receptor antagonists and phosphodiesterase 5 inhibitors.

Digoxin

Digoxin is often prescribed at a low dose more for its inotropic effect than as an antiarrhythmic. Despite being prescribed in up to half of all patients with pulmonary hypertension, the evidence basis is weak. A small RCT from 1981 in cor pulmonale (Group 3) patients did show an improvement in right ventricular function after 8 weeks but only when in the context of biventricular dysfunction [52].

Acute administration of digoxin at time of right heart catheterisation shows physiological improvement in idiopathic PAH. There is haemodynamic improvement, namely a 10 % increase in cardiac output with no change in pulmonary vascular resistance, and also a reduction in circulating levels of noradrenaline [53]. There is however no long term data supporting the use of digoxin in pulmonary hypertension.

Beta Blockers

Beta-blockers have been considered relatively contraindicated in pulmonary arterial hypertension due to the negative inotropic and chronotropic effects impacting on right ventricular function. Due to the inability to increase stroke volume, the PH cardiac output in exercise is predominantly rate dependent [54].

In addition beta-blockers may cause pulmonary vasoconstriction as suggested by animal models. However 12 % of group 1 patients were taking beta-blockers in the REVEAL registry [55].

Contrary to the above, more recent evidence suggests beta-blockade may be safe in PAH. First beta-blockers were found to reverse right ventricular remodelling and improve function and cardiac output in a rat model [56]. A prospective controlled cohort of 94 patients of group 1 PAH patients revealed no statistical difference in clinical end-points including mortality and right sided heart failure [57].

Their prescription needs to be weighed up with the strength of indication. For example all group 2 patients should be on beta-blockers as optimisation of their left sided heart failure [58].

One problematic situation is propranolol used as secondary prophylaxis for oesophageal varices due to liver cirrhosis. Intuitively risk-benefit analysis would point towards treatment (ie. prevention of life-threatening haemorrhage) but evidence from a 10 patient prospective, uncontrolled study in PH associated with portal hypertension (group 1.4.3) showed that withdrawal of beta-blockers improved both functional status and cardiac output without adverse incident [59]. There were no variceal bleeds off beta-blockers over 1½ years, although 60 % with large varices at time of endoscopy were prophylactically banded before discontinuation.

Anti-arrhythmics

Restoration of sinus rhythm (whenever possible) is the best therapeutic strategy for atrial arrhythmias. This is due to the optimisation of haemaodynamics and is especially true for congenital heart disease patients given how poorly tolerated atrial arrhythmias can be. Hence amiodarone, electrical cardioversion and/or electrophysiology studies with ablation are frequently used.

Atrial fibrillation appears to be the most malignant and treatment resistant. One retrospective study of 231 patients with pulmonary arterial hypertension and medically treated CTEPH over 6 years identified 31 episodes of atrial tachyarrhythmia. Sinus rhythm was restored in all atrial flutter patients (n of 12, 3 of which were ablated) but in only 2 out of 13 atrial fibrillation.

Cumulative mortality was 82 % in rate controlled atrial fibrillation compared with 6.3 % when sinus rhythm was restored [60]. Contrary to left heart disease, ventricular arrhythmias appear to be less problematic.

The ESC/ERS guidelines do state digoxin "may be considered" as a rate-controlling strategy for atrial tachyarrhytmias [47].

Diuretics

Over half of all pulmonary hypertension patients are prescribed diuretics and there is undoubtedly symptomatic improvement in the context of right ventricular failure and fluid overload. There is no evidence behind their usage and RCTs will not be forthcoming due the ethics of a placebo arm.

Consequently current best practice, as suggested by the ESC guidelines, is an individualised, clinical decision in the hands of the physician regarding choice, dose and timing of any diuretic therapy, taking into account renal function and serum potassium level [47].

Oxygen

The best evidence for supplemental oxygen therapy comes from the hypoxaemic, group 3 patient population, predominantly COPD. Long term oxygen therapy (LTOT) was proven to confer a survival advantage in hypoxaemic COPD (especially with signs of PH) patients over 30 years ago [61, 62].

In COPD associated PH, LTOT has been shown to improve mean PA pressure at repeat right heart catheterisation by 4.1 mmHg over 19 months [63]. It does appear that approximately only 60 % respond to oxygen therapy and this group has a marked mortality benefit (88 % 2 year survival compared with 22 %) [64].

Hence the ESC guidelines for all PH suggest following the COPD guidelines (most recently reaffirmed by NICE in 2010 [65, 66], namely long term oxygen therapy (used for at least 15 h a day) when resting p_aO_2 is less than 8.0 kPa [47].

40 % of PAH patients in the REVEAL registry were on LTOT [55]. Nocturnal desaturation is likely to be common even in the IPAH group (77 % in this 2001 study of 13 patients, predicted by resting p_aO^2, exertional desaturation and impaired spirometry/gas transfer) [67]. Therefore even in the absence of sleep disordered breathing, consideration should be given to overnight oximetry. Nocturnal oxygen therapy in PH has not been studied (except for Eisenmenger's syndrome) but keeping oxygen saturations above 90 % seems sensible.

Exercise

There is a growing body of evidence that supervised rehabilitation programmes are beneficial in PH. The putative mechanism is not dissimilar to skeletal muscle weakness as in COPD. First examined by prospective cross-over trial in 2006 showed a 22 % improvement in 6 min walk test after 15 weeks. There was also statistically significant improvement in functional class, quality of life questionnaires and VO_2 max. Due to safety concerns the exercise regimen was commenced whilst participants were hospital inpatients but there were no adverse events witnessed. There was not any difference in echocardiographic measurements [68].

Such symptomatic improvement has been reproduced in several studies over a range of aetiologies and supervised graded exercise appears safe even at the severe end of disease spectrum [69–71].

Specific Aetiologies

Anorexigen Induced (Nice Group 1.3)

Several of the targeted vasodilator studies included PAH secondary to anorexigen usage and it seems to behave in a not dissimilar fashion to IPAH [72] and hence its treatment follows suit. One difference is a slightly higher response rate to vasoreactivity testing (and hence calcium channel blocker use), 13.4 % in one study [73].

Connective Tissue Disease (Nice Group 1.4.1)

As above, connective tissue disease (CTD) associated PH was often included in the targeted vasodilator studies and hence its treatment algorithm mirrors that of IPAH [47]. It is however generally believed that the CTD cases respond less well to vasodilators than IPAH and often subgroup analyses of the above landmark trials failed to reach significance.

The strongest body of evidence comes from endothelin receptor antagonists and this uncontrolled trial of bosentan in all CTD PH revealed an improvement in functional class in 27 % [74].

There is one RCT with system sclerosis which showed an improved 6MWT on intravenous epoprostenol [75].

Systemic lupus erythematous and mixed connective tissue disorder patients with milder PH (FC I, II or III with a cardiac index of more than 3.1 l/mi/m²) appear to benefit from immunospressive therapy alone (cyclophosphamide and corticosteroids) [76].

Although there is a degree of vasoreactivity at right heart catheterisation, CTD related PH patients do not respond longer term to calcium channel blockers and consequently their use should be avoided. One postulated mechanism is the increased incidence of veno-occlusion, giving a PVOD like picture [73, 77]. Care needs to be given to anticoagulation due to the higher incidence of bleeding diatheses.

Human Immunodeficiency Virus (Nice Group 1.4.2)

Patients with Human Immunodeficiency Virus (HIV) have an increased risk of PAH development which increases their morbidity and mortality. The pathogenesis may involve a direct insult from the virus itself causing endothelial dysfunction in the lung vasculature, with the HIV Nef protein implicated in several studies [78]. PAH can develop in patients with well controlled HIV infection, on or off antiretroviral therapy.

Patients with confirmed HIV associated PAH are treated with antiretroviral therapy and stabilisation or improvement in pulmonary haemodynamics has been reported [79–81]. In the majority of cases advanced pulmonary vasodilator therapy is also commenced following diagnosis. This decision is made according to the patient's symptoms and other prognostic factors including their PVR, with careful prospective monitoring to ensure treatments are initiated and escalated when appropriate. Patients in WHO functional class III and IV are routinely offered both therapies at diagnosis.

Drug interactions between antiretroviral therapy and advanced pulmonary vasodilator therapies are important in patient management. HIV protease inhibitors mediate Cytochrome P450 isoenzyme inhibition. This markedly increases the levels of phosphodiesterase inhibitors as they are metabolised by Cytochrome P450 [82]. Sildenafil is mainly metabolised by Cytochrome P450 and a safe and effective dose for its concurrent use with protease inhibitors has not been established and its use is therefore contraindicated. If used, therapeutic drug monitoring is necessary [83]. The US Food and Drug Administration advise that when patients are taking protease inhibitors to instead start tadalafil when clinically necessary at a reduced dose of 20 mg once daily, increased to 40 mg once daily based upon individual tolerability.

Endothelin receptor antagonists (ERA) are also metabolised in the liver by Cytochrome P450 and therefore when prescribed with protease inhibitors, elevated ERA plasma concentrations can result [84, 85]. When prescribing bosentan in combination with protease inhibitors dose reductions are therefore recommended at 62.5 mg once daily or every other day [86]. There is less potential for increased ambrisentan levels when taking protease inhibitors and therefore only careful clinical monitoring is deemed appropriate with no dose change necessary. Co-administration of bosentan and the protease inhibitor atazanavir (Reyataz) without ritonavir is not recommended as the level of atazanavir is significantly reduced by the Cytochrome P450 isoenzyme inductive effects of bosentan (unlike ambrisentan) [87]. This has not been demonstrated with other protease inhibitors.

Bosentan has been successfully used as advanced pulmonary vasodilator therapy in HIV associated PAH [81, 88, 89] including 5 % of patients in the EARLY study bosentan treatment arm [11]. Other pulmonary vasodilator therapies that have been successfully used in the treatment of HIV associated PAH include intravenous epoprostenol [90–92], subcutaneous trepostinil [93] and inhaled iloprost [94]. Significant drug interactions with antiretroviral agents are not anticipated with these therapies. The use of combination therapies in patients with HIV associated PAH have only been published as single cases [81] and in positive RCTs inclusive of but not powered to investigate HIV subpopulations [38, 41, 42].

Data relating to the treatment of HIV associated PAH is limited and the management of patients is not well established. Treatment choices are influenced by the potential interactions between advanced pulmonary vasodilator treatments and co-administered anti-retroviral agents. Especially at the beginning of combined treatment, patients are carefully monitored for evidence of drug toxicity, with regular clinical review. In our current practice we routinely commence tadalafil as first line targeted treatment in HIV associated PAH, at the lower dose advised if on a concurrent protease inhibitor. If dual advanced pulmonary vasodilator treatment is appropriate we would then commence an ERA at the advised dose.

Portal Hypertension (Nice Group 1.4.3)

Pulmonary hypertension secondary to liver disease occurs only in the context of portal hypertension. The overall prevalence of PAH in portal hypertension is 2 % [95] and up to

8.5 % in the most severely affected population awaiting liver transplantation [96]. It is important to note that porto-pulmonary hypertension is a very distinct clinical entity from hepatopulmonary syndrome which is caused by microscopic arteriovenous malformations and lowers PVR.

The exact pathophysiology of porto-pulmonary hypertension has not been elucidated but is believed to be due one or more vasoactive cytokines (for example endothelin-1) bypassing their usual metabolism in the liver via porto-systemic shunting and directly impacting on the pulmonary vascular bed [97]. Histological findings are identical to IPAH. In addition to vasoconstriction, contributing factors likely include smooth muscle proliferation, in situ thrombosis, thromboembolism and a hyperdynamic circulation.

The same IPAH treatment algorithm for advanced therapy is followed but the evidence basis is less strong [47]. There are observational studies with each class of advanced vasodilator showing efficacy [98–100]. Consideration needs to be given to the vasodilatory impact on the portal circulation with prostacyclin analogues reported to cause increased flow and progressive splenomegaly [101]. Despite the adverse effect of hepatic dysfunction with endothelin receptor anatgonists, they do appear safe to use [102].

One difference is that vasoreactivity testing need not be performed as calcium channel blockers would not be used due to their effect on systemic vascular resistance. Anticoagulation is not advised due to the coagulopathy and the (especially variceal) bleeding risk. Beta blockers are discussed above.

Historically porto-pulmonary hypertension was considered an absolute contra-indication to liver transplantation. This is no longer the case, especially with mild disease, and there are case reports of PH resolving post-transplantation [103]. However outcomes are worse with more advanced PH [96]. Advanced vasodilators (usually intravenous prostanoids) are frequently employed in the perioperative period.

In terms of patients with co-existent liver dysfunction and pulmonary hypertension of another cause, care is needed with the choice of targeted vasodilator. Ambrisentan is preferred over bosentan but a PDE5 inhibitor would be first-line. Close monitoring of liver function tests is necessary.

Congenital Heart Disease (Nice Group 1.4.4)

Most severely affected (and well-studied) in congenital heart disease associated PH are those in whom Eisenmenger's syndrome has developed (elevated pressures causing reversal of flow via intra-cardiac shunt or patent ductus arteriosis). Historically considered untreatable, vasodilators have shown to improve clinical and haemodynamic outcomes [104].

Bosentan carries the most weight of evidence. Some non-Eisenmenger congenital heart disease patients were included in the EARLY trial [11]. The BREATHE-5 trial showed good efficacy of bosentan in terms of function and haemodynamics with FC III over 16 and 40 weeks (placebo RCT and open label respectively) [105]. In addition, by having similar impact on pulmonary and systemic vascular resistance, there was no worsening of shunt and hence oxygenation was maintained.

There is unblinded prospective evidence for sildenafil that it can also improve oxygenation levels as well as functioning [106, 107].

Advanced vasodilators also carry a reduction in all-cause mortality as seen with the Royal Brompton Hospital's cohort of 229 Eisenmenger's patients. The majority were talking bosentan and were followed-up for several years [108].

Anticoagulation is an individualised risk-benefit decision given both thrombotic tendency (reduced pulmonary flow, secondary erythrocytosis) and haemorrhagic complications (haemoptysis, cerebrovascular) seen in this population. Calcium channel blockers should not be prescribed as they can worsen the right to left shunt with disastrous consequences. Despite being contrary to common sense, nocturnal oxygen does not appear to have any effect [109] and long term oxygen therapy is only recommended if there is improvement if terms of symptoms and oxygenation. Aggressive correction of arrhythmias is particularly important.

Schistosomiasis (Nice Group 1.4.5)

Schistosomiasis may be the commonest cause of PH worldwide but, other than antiparasitic agents, its best treatment is completely unknown. It is caused by infection with the trematode (blood fluke) parasite *Schistosoma* and affects over 200 million people worldwide. 7.7 % of those with chronic hepatosplenic schistosomiasis have pulmonary hypertension at RHC [110]. Transmission is through contaminated water with freshwater snails the intermediate hosts and it is endemic in wide areas of Africa, Asia, the Middle East and South America.

Of the three commonest species of the parasite, two especially (*Schistosoma mansoni and japonicum*) cause pulmonary hypertension. The larval form enters through the skin and travel through the circulation to the liver and intestine. After 2 months' maturation, eggs are produced and deposit in the pulmonary vascular bed, both causing mechanical obstruction and a granulomatous endarteritis through inflammatory cytokine secretion. Portal hypertension also contributes to the pathophysiology.

Given the high prevalence of schistosomiasis and the likelihood of re-infection post treatment, public health strategies have focused more on prevention, especially the provision of clean water and snail control. Praziquantel is the first-line antihelminthic and effective as a single dose, however does not appear to improve the haemodynamics [110]. The advanced vasodilators have not been well studied and given the global distribution of the disease and the large costs entailed it does unfortunately seem unlikely that they will be in the near future. There is some very limited evidence (essentially case reports) behind sildenafil's use [111, 112].

One uncontrolled, observational study on 12 patients using either phosphodiesterase-5 inhibitor or endothelin receptor antagonist showed a FC and 6MWT improvement [113].

Pulmonary Veno-occlusive Disease (Nice Group 1')

Vasodilators carry a higher risk in pulmonary veno-occlusive disease (PVOD) as being selective for the arterial side there is the chance of pulmonary oedema developing secondary to hydrostatic capillary pressure. There have been fatalities reported with IV epoprostenol [114]. In specialised centres, prostanoids may be commenced safely when done very cautiously and they appear to be efficacious [115, 116].

There is no data with endothelin receptor antagonists or phosphodiesterase-5 inhibitors. Warfarin, oxygen and early referral for lung transplantation are usually considered. There are case reports of immunosuppressive medication (in this case steroids and azathioprine) being used in the context of autoimmune features [117].

Left Heart Disease (Nice Group 2)

The primary therapy of group 2 PH is optimisation of the heart failure [58]. This is the same for heart failure with reduced and preserved left ventricular systolic function and secondary to valvular disease. Reducing left ventricular end-diastolic pressure reduces the passive transmitted PH. ACE inhibitors and beta blockers are the mainstay and neither are contraindicated in PH.

There have been a number of trials of advanced vasodilators in heart failure without much benefit seen and significant adverse events [118, 119]. Currently they are not recommended but trials are ongoing. Sildenafil carries some supporting data predominantly in terms of improved haemodynamics [120, 121].

Chronic Obstructive Pulmonary Disease (Nice Group 3.1)

The mainstay of treatment for all Dana point group 3 patients (lung diseases and/or hypoxia) is, as the name implies, oxygenation. The evidence for oxygen in COPD associated PH is discussed in the previous section. In summary there is improvement of PA pressures but not reversal to normality.

Early observational evidence suggested a role for targeted vasodilators in PH secondary to lung disease, sildenafil especially [122]. However they are of limited use due to the deleterious side-effect of worsening oxygenation. Despite acutely improving haemodynamics, they have the significant downside of worsening of ventilation/perfusion mismatch. This is secondary to deregulation of the hypoxic pulmonary vasoconstriction mechanism. Hence any potential benefit is offset by worsening of the hypoxaemia that is driving the pulmonary hypertension. A cut-off point of FEV1 60 % predicted is sometimes used as a complete contraindication.

In COPD specifically, sildenafil has been shown to improve haemodynamics but this is countered by worsening degree of hypoxaemia [123]. This blinded RCT of sildenafil in COPD did show an improvement in 6MWT [124]. Results for bosentan in COPD have been mixed [125].

Intriguingly, pravastatin has been shown by RCT to improve exercise capacity and pulmonary vascular resistance in COPD associated PH [126]. The proposed mechanism is inhibition of endothelin-1 production.

Severe PH not explained by the severity of lung disease (the recently discarded concept of "out of proportion" disease) is more worthy of advance vasodilator treatment due to the possibility of additional pathophysiological processes. If the mean PA pressure is over 40 mmHg then referral onto specialist centre for consideration of vasodilators may be warranted.

Interstitial Lung Disease (Nice Group 3.2)

The supplemental oxygen guidelines are as those for COPD, although this has not been investigated on a stand-alone basis. Concerns about worsening mismatch with targeted vasodilators are equally prominent.

Sildenafil once again has the most support although the evidence basis is limited. Both sildenafil and epoprostenol acutely lower PVR but gas exchange actually improved with sildenafil maybe by acting more locally and hence enhancing ventilation-perfusion matching [127].

Nebulised iloprost is the preferred prostanoid (with presumed less systemic effects impacting on hypoxic pulmonary vasoconstriction) with demonstrated improvement in function, symptoms and haemodynamics [128]. Intravenous epoprostenol worsens gas exchange and hence increases hypoxaemia.

There is no place for the use of endothelin receptor antagonists. Bosentan is not efficacious in idiopathic pulmonary fibrosis or systemic sclerosis associated ILD as seen by the placebo controlled RCTs [129–131]. Ambrisentan in the ARIES-3 study actually reduced 6MWT by 23 m in ILD associated PH (as it also did to a lesser extent in COPD) [14].

This was supported and made even more concerning by ARTEMIS-IPF which was terminated early after recruiting 492 idiopathic pulmonary fibrosis patients. Of note only 10 % of the study group had PH. The ambrisentan treatment arm showed statistically significant disease progression and more hospitalisation episodes compared with placebo. There was also non-significant higher mortality of 7.9 % compared with 3.7 % (p of 0.10) [9].

Sleep Disordered Breathing (Nice Group 3.4)

Continuous positive airways pressure treating obstructive sleep apnoea has been shown to reduce pulmonary artery pressure in a well-designed cross-over trial using sham CPAP (subtherapeutic positive end-expiratory pressure) as the control arm [132]. Repeat polysomnography on nocturnal CPAP therapy is indicated to ensure the apnoea-hypopnoea index and level of oxygenation is acceptable.

In the context of PH secondary to obesity hypoventilation syndrome then non-invasive ventilation plus/minus oxygen therapy is likely to be needed and beneficial to the PH but has not been directly studied.

Weight loss is highly important but often difficult to achieve. The wide health benefits of bariatric surgery include significant reduction in mean PA pressures [133].

There is no evidence to support the use of targeted vasodilator medication in sleep disordered breathing associated PH.

Chronic Thromboembolic Disease (Nice Group 4)

Pulmonary thromboendarterectomy for chronic thromboembolic pulmonary hypertension (CTEPH) is discussed in the next chapter. There remains a role for advanced vasodilators as a bridge to surgery and in those not amenable to surgical intervention (for example with distal thromboembolic disease or co-morbidities precluding such major surgery) [134].

Medical therapy results in only limited improvement and, unlike surgery, is in no way curative. Bosentan is the best researched and the BENEFiT placebo RCT showed a 22 % reduction in PVR but no benefit in terms of exercise capacity [135]. A 2010 metanalysis of 10 (mainly open label, uncontrolled) bosentan studies showed significant but modest improvements in 6MWT and PA pressure [136]. Ambrisentan increased the mean 6MWT by 17 m and reduced BNP by 22 % in 28 uncontrolled, proximal and distal CTEPH patients [14].

Prostacyclin analogues and phosphodiesterase-5 inhibtors do also have some supporting evidence [137–140]. Riociguat has also been investigated with promising results in this group and more detail is given below.

The use of vasodilators as a bridge to surgery is only done at the severe end of the spectrum with evidence of right ventricular dysfunction. FC III and IV patients with high a PVR (over 15 Wood units) have been tested with intravenous epoprostenol. This revealed haemodynamic improvement and a postoperative mortality of 8.3 % that (although far higher than those with less severe disease) compared favourably with other studies in similarly advanced patients [141]. There is a evidence against the need for routine use pre-operatively [142].

The final patient group in whom medical therapy is considered are those with persisting PH post pulmonary endarterectomy. There is limited evidence but the BENEFiT trial included this group and they comprised 28 % of the cohort [135]. Despite PH persisting at the 3 month mark postoperatively, when advanced vasodilators are commenced, there is no increased mortality for at least 4 years compared with those who responded well [143].

Sickle Cell Disease (Nice Group 5.1)

Previously in group 1, the haemolytic anaemias including sickle cell have been moved to group 5 following the 2013 world symposium in Nice [144]. The results with targeted vasodilators in sickle cell disease related PH have been disappointing. There is pathophysiological rationale for using phosphodiesterase-5 inhibitors, given the lack of NO bioavailability in its pathogenesis, but sildenafil has shown a high rate of complications, specifically vaso-occlusive crises [145].

L-arginine, a precursor of NO, given orally, produces an acute reduction in PA pressures (by a mean of 15 %) [146].

Sarcoidosis (Nice Group 5.2)

Corticosteroids are the mainstay of treatment for many of the manifestations of sarcoidosis. The evidence for their use in pulmonary hypertension is mixed. This likely reflects the multifactorial pathophysiology. One retrospective study suggests that the steroid response is only seen in the absence of pulmonary fibrosis [147].

Targeted vasodilators do have case studies suggesting efficacy but RCTs are awaited. Complicating matters is the heterogeneity of clinical manifestation and hence extrapolation within subsets. Caution is required with vasodilator commencement due to the worsening of gas exchange (as per other causes of ILD), pulmonary oedema (with post-capillary disease similar to PVOD) and myocardial involvement [148].

Intravenous epoprostenol demonstrated haemodynamic and functional response but with the risk of complication [149]. Sildenafil and bosentan have both been shown to significantly improve pulmonary haemodynamics but not benefit 6MWT [150, 151].

Contrary to corticosteroids, those with fibrotic lung disease may benefit more (especially if the fibrosis is milder) and this retrospective review of different classes of vasodilators did demonstrate an improvement in 6MWT [152].

Special Circumstances

Air Travel

Air travel is a convenient method of transport but exposes passengers with cardiorespiratory disease to potentially hazardous conditions. Although aircraft cabins are pressurised, cabin air pressure at cruising altitude is still lower than air pressure at sea level at an equivalent altitude of 1800–2400 m above sea level. The reduced barometric pressure determines a reduced partial pressure of oxygen in ambient air and this results in a degree of hypoxia for travellers. The normal physiological response to low alveolar oxygen is pulmonary arterial vasoconstriction. The response to prolonged hypoxia in PH patients in flight is unpredictable but can lead to a degree of pulmonary vasoconstriction that increases

PVR. Allied to this, air travel is associated with relative dehydration and extended immobility increasing thromboembolic risk, and air recirculation in a confined environment risking cross infection. The condition of patients with PH is typically only stable within narrow limits and therefore any increase in PVR can result in a patient's condition deteriorating exponentially in flight.

There is a distinct lack of evidence and no strict guidelines recommending the safety of flying or suitable pre-flight assessments in PH patients. The 2008 ESC/ERS guidelines [47] suggest that consideration should be given to the use of in-flight oxygen for patients in WHO functional class 3 or 4. Patients with arterial oxygen concentration consistently below 8 kPa are considered for long-term oxygen therapy and these patients should continue therapy in flight. The British Thoracic Society air travel guidelines 2011 [153] support these recommendations and do not advocate routine hypoxic challenge testing.

We would encourage careful consideration on an individual level, for any patient with PH who wishes to fly. This should incorporate an assessment of symptom severity, haemodynamic impairment (PVR) and the degree of hypoxia pre travel. Any concurrent diseases associated with PH or separate to their PH diagnosis which may be adversely affected by air travel should also be incorporated into this assessment.

In general we would suggest that if resting oxygen saturation levels are above 92 % on room air and the patient is WHO functional class I or II then supplementary oxygen therapy may not be required in flight. For all other PH patients we would recommend up to date arterial blood gas analysis to accurately determine their arterial oxygen concentration at sea level. Supplementary oxygen should then be prescribed appropriately (to achieve arterial oxygen saturation of >8kPa) for the duration of the flight.

Our centre performs formal fitness to fly assessments for patients that require long term oxygen therapy and who are in WHO functional class III and IV. We also refer patients for these assessments if they have previously had adverse symptoms in flight. If a patient does not fulfil the criteria for long term oxygen therapy on blood gas analysis then 15 % inspired oxygen concentration (FiO2) is delivered via an occlusive mask with a one way valve for twenty minutes. If the measured arterial oxygen concentration is below 6.6 kPa then supplemental oxygen is prescribed as standard in flight. In order to discern the appropriate supplementary oxygen delivery rate for patients requiring oxygen therapy in flight, supplemental oxygen is delivered via nasal cannulae inside a body box containing 15 % FiO_2. Blood gas analysis is not possible inside the body box, instead peripheral oxygen saturation level and transcutaneous carbon dioxide monitoring are used. The delivery rate of supplemental oxygen is titrated up until a peripheral saturation level above 85 % is achieved. Provided that patients do not become unwell or develop hypercapnia during testing they are then prescribed oxygen in flight at the delivery rate identified. Most patients require a delivery rate of 2 L/min if they do not require long term oxygen therapy at sea level. If a patient has high PVR and /or high oxygen requirements at sea level or during fitness to fly assessment, then we do not recommend air travel on medical grounds given the unpredictable potential dangers the situation imposes.

In patients with congenital heart disease associated PAH, oxygen would not be predicted to improve the arterial oxygen saturation due to the presence of significant intracardiac shunting. Patients in WHO functional class I and II may often travel by air without the need for supplemental oxygen therapy or fitness to fly assessment.

It is important that all PH patients understand the unpredictable risk involved in air travel. Patients must be aware of the individual airlines policy regarding in-flight oxygen and contact the airline in plenty of time to inform them of their requirements. When abroad, all PH patients should have written information available describing their condition(s) and know who to contact in the case of deteriorating health.

Pregnancy

Many patients with PH are of child bearing age. During pregnancy and postpartum many physiological changes occur which present a significant risk for patients with PH. In normal pregnancy, circulating blood volume expands by 30–50 %, which is maximal between 28 and 34 weeks gestation and largely due to increased plasma volume. This increases cardiac preload and hence stroke volume and cardiac output. An increase in resting heart rate also contributes to increasing cardiac output. Cardiac output progressively rises from the first trimester to reach up to 150 % of pre-pregnancy levels. Systemic vasodilatation also occurs during pregnancy and together with the presence of a low resistance placental circulation drops systemic vascular resistance. This can result in a fall in systemic blood pressure. During labour, cardiac output increases by a further 25–50 %. This is partly due to greater intravascular blood volume from the contracting uterus redirecting blood to expand circulating blood volume. Also, catecholamine secretion related to the pain and apprehension of labour increases cardiac output. After delivery, the inferior vena cava is decompressed and uterine blood again increases circulating volume, cardiac filling pressure and cardiac output. Only 6 weeks after delivery do the cardiovascular physiological changes associated with pregnancy approach normal pre-pregnancy levels [154, 155].

The right ventricle and the pulmonary circulation receive the entire cardiac output but can ordinarily adapt to accommodate variable loading conditions. The chronic elevation in PVR in patients with PH can result in right ventricular dysfunction with tricuspid regurgitation from ventricular dilatation and predisposition to arrhythmia. Remodelling in the pulmonary circulation also limits the ability to adapt to variable blood flow. It is therefore predictable that the significant haemodynamic changes associated with pregnancy and peripartum are poorly tolerated. PAH patients may not be able to endure the increased blood volume and heart rate demanded by pregnancy and labour. They are at risk of circulatory collapse, therapy resistant right heart failure and arrhythmia. The PVR may rise acutely, reducing venous return to the left side of the heart with profound systemic hypotension, termed PAH crisis. All of these situations can be fatal.

The hypercoagulable state in pregnancy and particularly post-partum is also a concern in PAH patients. Any thromboembolic event afflicting the already compromised pulmonary vasculature can be life threatening. Similarly, stroke may result from paradoxical embolism when intracardiac shunting is present [156].

The evidence supporting management decisions for patients in pregnancy with PAH is limited to individual reports and case series. However it is universally acknowledged that multidisciplinary input and close monitoring throughout pregnancy is central to a successful outcome [157]. The multidisciplinary team must meet regularly and include a high-risk obstetric anaesthetic team with experience in PH. We also advocate that patients should have at least monthly echocardiograms and clinical review by a PH specialist through their pregnancy. Admission to hospital for monitoring is advocated when approaching labour or with any clinical deterioration. Supportive care includes fluid regimes, diuretics, appropriate oxygen therapy, advanced pulmonary vasodilator therapies and inotropic support when necessary.

Sildenafil is often given as first line advanced pulmonary vasodilator therapy in pregnancy [158–161]. Sildenafil causes uterine artery vasodilation and is also used in the treatment of pre-term and term neonatal PH [162]. Alternatively, or if there is any clinical deterioration, prostanoids such as illoprost [157, 163, 164] or epoprostenol are prescribed [165, 166]. There have also been positive reports using oral calcium channel blockers [167, 168]. Inhaled NO may cause an acute drop in PVR when given, in Eisenmenger syndrome [169], idiopathic PAH [170] and CTEPH [171], and has been successfully used in pregnancy [172, 173]. Endothelin receptor antagonists are

118   A. Loveridge et al.

contra-indicated in pregnancy due to animal studies showing possible teratogenic effects [174]. Women of child bearing age are notified of this prior to commencing therapy and alternative classes of advanced pulmonary vasodilator therapy are used. In our centre, all patients with PH on oral advanced pulmonary vasodilator therapies that are planning pregnancy or become pregnant are converted to sildenafil treatment when possible. If increased disease modifying therapy is necessary then patients are commenced on intravenous prostanoid treatment. Anticoagulation is considered in pregnancy in patients with PH but must be carefully controlled when nearing delivery [175].

Planned elective births are advised [47]. Less patients are undergoing vaginal birth and more patients are undergoing planned premature deliveries in the modern management era [157, 175]. For most patients we advocate an elective planned delivery using caesarean section and regional anaesthesia, avoiding the adverse haemodynamic consequences of labour, which may be prolonged. Patients receiving general anaesthesia appear to have higher mortality compared to the use of regional anaesthesia (odds ratio 3.7) [175]. There is however no consensus regarding the mode and timing of delivery in PAH parturients. Maternal safety needs to be compared to the risk of premature delivery, intrauterine growth restriction and the need for neonatal care input.

There is evidence to suggest that with better knowledge and multidisciplinary management in pregnancy, improved outcomes have been achieved in pregnant patients with PAH. A systematic review of published outcomes of pregnancy in PAH and CTEPH compared reported mortality from 1978 to 1996 [176] with results from 1997 to 2007. Mortality decreased from 30 to 17 % in idiopathic PAH, 36–28 % in congenital heart disease associated PAH and from 56 to 33 % in other groups. Seventy eight percent of maternal deaths occurred within the first month following delivery [175]. Neonatal or foetal death occurred in 10 % of cases and intrauterine growth restriction was reported in 18 % of pregnancies [175]. Notably publication bias towards a positive outcome may have artificially lowered published figures in both review periods. There appears to be no statistically significant difference in maternal or foetal outcome between different subgroups of patients with PAH or CTEPH [175].

Despite improving experience and outcomes, pregnancy is associated with significant mortality in PAH and CTEPH patients. Thirty percent of pregnancies in women with PAH occur in patients who were not aware of their disease prior to pregnancy [177]. However, many patients diagnosed with PH are of childbearing age and early discussions regarding the risks of pregnancy are mandatory. This ensures an informed decision is made and suitable contraception is prescribed as appropriate. Bosentan may reduce the efficacy of regular oral contraceptive agents as it induces cytochrome P450 enzymes. Therefore alternative contraceptive methods are used if this drug is given to patients of child bearing age. Levonorgestrel can be taken within 72 h to terminate pregnancy if chosen but the dose must be doubled if given to patients taking bosentan.

Renal Failure

Patients with chronic or end stage renal disease have a high prevalence of PH owing to unclear multifactorial pathophysiology that remains poorly understood. They therefore are placed in group 5 of the clinical classification of PH. No specific intervention trial aimed at reducing PH in patients with chronic kidney disease has been performed to date. Correcting volume overload and treating left ventricular disorders are important in this patient population. When clinically appropriate, treatment with advanced pulmonary vasodilator therapy is however routinely commissioned for patients in the UK with PH associated with chronic renal failure using dialysis [4].

Patients with PH from any cause may develop acute or chronic renal impairment. According to the British National Formulary the following advanced pulmonary vasodilator therapies should be modified within the context of renal impairment. Consideration should be given to a reduction in the prescribed dose frequency of sildenafil if the drug is not tolerated in renal failure, from three times daily to twice daily, especially when the estimated glomerular filtration rate is below 30 ml/min/1.73 m^2. The starting dose of tadalafil should be halved in mild to moderate renal impairment and titrated up to full dose as tolerated. Ambrisentan should be used with caution when the estimated glomerular filtration rate is below 30 ml/min/1.73 m^2.

Assessment and Peri-operative Management of Patients with Pulmonary Hypertension

It is essential that patients with pulmonary hypertension who are being considered for elective surgery attend a pre-operative anaesthetic/high risk clinic and for the clinicians involved to have close contact with those working in the pulmonary hypertension centre. It is important to be aware of the patient's baseline state, their predicated life expectancy without the proposed surgical intervention, the complications which may arise and what treatment strategies should be put in place if the patient is unable to take their usual oral maintenance therapy. Additional attention (in conjunction with the surgeon) will be given to the type of operation performed. For example for some patients laparoscopic abdominal surgery may not be possible as the patient would be poorly tolerant of the adverse haemodynamic and cardiothoracic physiological impacts of abdominal gas insufflation causing reducing venous return and reducing lung volumes and adversely affecting lung perfusion, pulmonary vascular resistance and gas exchange capabilities. Finally if the patient has other co-morbidities or if the pulmonary hypertension is part of a multisystem disease then consultation with other specialists involved in the patient's management should be sought. It may be considered appropriate for the patient to have their surgery in the pulmonary hypertension centre although this is not always possible as many of these centres are primarily cardiothoracic and will not necessarily have the infrastructure to look after patients with pulmonary hypertension who have other pathologies or require other forms of surgical intervention. Patients with congenital heart disease should have all their management undertaken whenever possible in the congenital heart disease centre.

It is often advisable for a cardiothoracic anaesthetist to be involved during the operative procedure. A perioperative pulmonary artery catheter is frequently deployed to help guide fluid resuscitation, monitor pulmonary vascular resistance and cardiac output and to diagnose and assess response to treatment should a pulmonary hypertension crisis arise. Post operatively patients are usually managed in a high dependency or intensive care unit. It is most important during the peri-opertive period that the patients systemic vascular resistance does not fall below the pulmonary vascular resistance as under such circumstances profound haemodynamic disturbance and death can occur. If patients are tolerant of ongoing oral therapy this may be given nasogastricaly assuming the patient is absorbing through this route. If oral therapy is not possible there are no routinely available intravenous alternative formulations for phosphodiesterase type 5 inhibitors and endothelin receptor antagonists and therefore other agents must be considered. These include nebulised or intravenous prostacyclin, nebulised nitric oxide or intravenous milrinone or vasopressin. Subcutaneous therapy may be unreliably absorbed particularly if the patient's circulation is compromised and if they are receiving inotropic support such as adrenaline or nor-adrenaline which may compromise skin perfusion. For those patients with congenital heart disease it is most important to continuously maintain the systemic vascular resistance above the pulmonary vascular resistance, to ensure that hydration is optimal and that there is close monitoring of haemoglobin and iron stores. Some patients may be candidates for intra-operative transesophageal echo cardio graphic monitoring.

Normal baseline advanced pulmonary vasodilative therapy is commenced as soon as possible after surgery. An early appointment with the pulmonary hypertension clinic will be made and appropriate follow up will continue possibly with ongoing surgical follow up appointments as indicated. Throughout the whole pathway, close communication between the health care professionals involved in the patients care is mandatory to ensure the best possible outcome.

Novel/Future Therapies

Despite the vast progress made in the field, pulmonary arterial hypertension still confers a high burden of functional impairment and remains a progressive, fatal condition. Targeted vasodilators have ameliorated the symptoms and improved life expectancy but only prolong the inevitable. Pulmonary thromboendarterectomy for CTEPH is the only potentially curative treatment. PH secondary to other conditions universally confers a worse prognosis and there is a far more limited understanding of therapeutic strategies with these groups.

There is no inclinication from the PH community to rest on its laurels [178]. Work continues apace to better understand the optimal use for those therapies we already have and develop new classes of medication. Multiple possible future therapies are already at the clinical trial stage. In addition to looking at other targets within the endothelin, NO and prostacyclin pathways, new candidate drugs are targeting the immune system and cellular proliferation with the ultimate goal of reverse remodelling. Some already have proven benefit whereas many others have had success in animal models but this has not transitioned into efficacious proof of concept trials in humans.

Riociguat

Soluble guanylate cyclase is the intracellular receptor for nitric oxide. Riociguat (BAY 63–2521) stimulates soluble guanylate cyclise both directly (mimicking NO) and by increasing its sensitivity to endogenous NO. This leads to cGMP augmentation with vasodilatation and anti-prolifera-tion. There are promising results in both PAH and CTEPH and it has just been licensed by the FDA but not yet by the MHRA. It has a good safety profile with infrequent syncope the main adverse effect.

Versus placebo in the PATENT-1 trial, riocigulat gave a highly significant increase in 6MWT of 36 m over 12 weeks. This involved 443 most PAH group patients, both treatment naive and already on ERAs or prostanoids and the benefit was seen regardless. Secondary endpoints of PVR, FC, dyspnoea, clinical worsening and BNP were also significantly improved on the highest dose [179]. The extension study PATENT-2 is in progress.

Building on phase 2 evidence in CTEPH was the recently reported CHEST-1. 261 inoperable or persistent CTEPH patients were involved in this placebo RCT. The 6MWT increased by 46 m and PVR decreased by 3 Wood units [180]. Again a long term extension in CHEST-2 is in progress.

Given such early promise, riociguat is also being investigated in other aetiologies of pulmonary hypertension. The RCT LEPHT looked at group 2 PH secondary to systolic dysfunc-tion. The primary endpoint of reduction in mean PA pressure was not met but there was significant improvement in both pulmonary vascular resistance and cardiac index [181]. There is also the suggestion of benefit in group 3 patient, namely ILD and COPD, in these small, open label studies [182, 183].

Cinaciguat is another guanylate cyclase activator with slightly different mechanism which is being developed for use in decom-pensated heart failure. It has only been studied in sheep models of persistent pulmonary hypertension of the newborn.

Selexipag

An efficacious oral prostanoid would be a big advance and selexipag has been developed as a prostacyclin receptor ago-nist that is showing far more promise than beraprost.

Selexipag and its active metabolite selectively target the prostaglandin I2 receptor (IP). Currently it is only at the proof of concept stage but a phase 3 randomised controlled trial, GRIPHON, should report in 2014. There is some phase 2 evidence that it is efficacious (with 30 % reduction in PVR and the non-significant 24 m increase in 6MWT) and is well tolerated [184].

Tyrosine Kinase Inhibitors

Receptor tyrosine kinases are cell surface receptors that trigger inflammatory cascades via phosphorylation. Important in the pathogenesis of pulmonary hypertension are those pathways of platelet derived growth factor (PDGF), vascular endothelial growth factor (VEGF), epidermal growth factor (EGF), insulin receptor (IR), fibroblast growth factor (FGF) and c-KIT with the end result of cellular proliferation and remodelling. Multiple tyrosine kinase inhibitors have been developed with marked success in the treatment of various cancers. They are exciting candidates for reverse remodelling in PH.

The IMPRES placebo RCT study looked at imatinib (targeting, amongst others, PDGF receptors) and has just resulted. The inclusion criteria were severe PAH patients despite already being on at least 2 advanced vasodilator medication. 202 patients were recruited and 6MWT increased by 32 m over 24 weeks (p of 0.002). These results were maintained at 48 weeks extension. There were also improvements in haemodynamics and BNP but neither functional class nor time to clinical worsening. Concerningly there were significantly more adverse events in the treatment arm (44 % versus 30 %), including 8 subdural haematomas on anticoagulation, and a high discontinuation rate [185].

Sorafenib acts on the VEGF receptor and is only at the phase 1 trial stage assessing safety in PAH [186]. Other tyrosine kinase inhibitors are being evaluated and developed.

Vasoactive Intestinal Peptide

Given vasoactive intestinal peptide's reduced concentration in PH and its effect on smooth muscle proliferation, it has been postulated as a therapy for PH. There was some early success in animal models but its promise has not been realised in humans and it has fallen by the wayside [187].

Adrenomedullin

Adrenomedullin is also a vasoactive peptide that was discovered in phaeochromcytomas. It cause vasodilatation and is associated with PAH disease severity. Inhaled, it causes acute benefit to haemodynamics at right heart catheterisation and cardiopulmonary exercise testing [188]. To date, studies have only been with single dose administration.

Fausdil

Rho-associated protein kinase (ROCK) is involved in smooth muscle contraction and remodelling. It is inhibited by fausdil which can be given via inhalation or intravenously. Inhaled it causes acute reduction in mean PA pressure and pulmonary vascular resistance equivalent to that of inhaled nictric oxide [189]. There is no longer term data.

Statins

Statins also inhibit the Rho pathway and there has been some success with their use in animal models and COPD associated PH [126]. However this benefit was not seen in PAH with several disappointing studies using simvastatin [190, 191].

Inhaled Nitric Oxide

Often used in the acute intensive care setting (in addition to vasoreactivity testing) with well documented haemodynamic effects, inhaled NO is now being evaluated as a chronic therapy. Currently the evidence is restricted to case reports and one series from the 1990s [192, 193] but a phase 2 trial in PAH as an add-on therapy is underway.

Cicletanine

Cicletanine is a diuretic that upregulates NO production (via coupling of endothelial nitric oxide synthase) and is used for systemic hypertension in Europe. By targeting endothelial dysfunction it is hoped that it may impact on PH's pathogenesis. The evidence behind it is currently limited to animals models and individual case studies [194]. Phase 2 trials are awaited.

Dichloroacetic Acid

Dichloroacetate is a chemical compound that affects the metabolic functioning of mitochrondria and has been researched in cancer. It reverses the remodelling of PH in rats and mice via increased apoptosis [195] but has not been studied in humans.

Terguride

Serotonin has a role in the pathogenesis of PH with remodelling effects on pulmonary artery fibroblasts and smooth muscle cells. Terguride is a partial dopamine D2, adrenergic and serotonin antagonist. It has anti-proliferative, anti-thrombotic and anti-fibrotic effects and causes relaxation of smooth muscle. Once again despite promising animal results, those in humans were disappointing [196].

Stem Cells

Circulating endothelial progenitor cells are involved with angiogenesis and remodelling and have been implicated in PAH pathogenesis with various reports of increased and decreased numbers [197].

Autologous transfusion of endothelial progenitor cells was useful in animal models and one prospective open label study in humans with IPAH. This showed a 42.5 m improvement in 6MWT plus improved haemodynamics [198].

Gene Therapy

BMPR2 gene therapy via adenovirus vector has been successful in a rat model of PH, improving haemodynamics and reducing vascular remodelling [199]. Given the difficulties experienced with gene therapy in other diseases, it remains only a distant possibility.

References

1. D'Alonzo GE, Barst RJ, Ayres SM, Bergofsky EH, Brundage BH, Detre KM, et al. Survival in patients with primary pulmonary hypertension. Results from a national prospective registry. Ann Intern Med. 1991;115(5):343–9.
2. Robin ED. The kingdom of the near-dead. The shortened unnatural life history of primary pulmonary hypertension. Chest. 1987;92(2):330–4.
3. Rich S, Kaufmann E, Levy PS. The effect of high doses of calcium-channel blockers on survival in primary pulmonary hypertension. N Engl J Med. 1992;327(2):76–81.
4. NHS Commissioning Board. Commissioning Policy Statement: National policy for targeted therapies for the treatment of pulmonary

hypertension in adults. March 2013. Available from: http://www.england.nhs.uk/wp-content/uploads/2013/04/a11-ps-a.pdf.

5. Galie N, Manes A, Negro L, Palazzini M, Bacchi-Reggiani ML, Branzi A. A meta-analysis of randomized controlled trials in pulmonary arterial hypertension. Eur Heart J. 2009;30(4): 394–403.

6. Benza RL, Miller DP, Barst RJ, Badesch DB, Frost AE, McGoon MD. An evaluation of long-term survival from time of diagnosis in pulmonary arterial hypertension from the REVEAL Registry. Chest. 2012;142(2):448–56.

7. Barst RJ, Langleben D, Badesch D, Frost A, Lawrence EC, Shapiro S, et al. Treatment of pulmonary arterial hypertension with the selective endothelin-A receptor antagonist sitaxsentan. J Am Coll Cardiol. 2006;47(10):2049–56.

8. Lavelle A, Sugrue R, Lawler G, Mulligan N, Kelleher B, Murphy DM, et al. Sitaxentan-induced hepatic failure in two patients with pulmonary arterial hypertension. Eur Respir J. 2009; 34(3):770–1.

9. Raghu G, Behr J, Brown KK, Egan JJ, Kawut SM, Flaherty KR, et al. Treatment of idiopathic pulmonary fibrosis with ambrisentan: a parallel, randomized trial. Ann Intern Med. 2013;158(9):641–9.

10. Rubin LJ, Badesch DB, Barst RJ, Galie N, Black CM, Keogh A, et al. Bosentan therapy for pulmonary arterial hypertension. N Engl J Med. 2002;346(12):896–903.

11. Galie N, Rubin L, Hoeper M, Jansa P, Al-Hiti H, Meyer G, et al. Treatment of patients with mildly symptomatic pulmonary arterial hypertension with bosentan (EARLY study): a double-blind, randomised controlled trial. Lancet. 2008;371(9630):2093–100.

12. Galie N, Olschewski H, Oudiz RJ, Torres F, Frost A, Ghofrani HA, et al. Ambrisentan for the treatment of pulmonary arterial hypertension: results of the ambrisentan in pulmonary arterial hypertension, randomized, double-blind, placebo-controlled, multicenter, efficacy (ARIES) study 1 and 2. Circulation. 2008;117(23):3010–9.

13. Oudiz RJ, Galie N, Olschewski H, Torres F, Frost A, Ghofrani HA, et al. Long-term ambrisentan therapy for the treatment of pulmonary arterial hypertension. J Am Coll Cardiol. 2009;54(21): 1971–81.

14. Badesch DB, Feldman J, Keogh A, Mathier MA, Oudiz RJ, Shapiro S, et al. ARIES-3: ambrisentan therapy in a diverse population of patients with pulmonary hypertension. Cardiovasc Ther. 2012;30(2):93–9.

15. Pulido T, Adzerikho I, Channick RN, Delcroix M, Galie N, Ghofrani HA, et al. Macitentan and morbidity and mortality in pulmonary arterial hypertension. N Engl J Med. 2013;369(9):809–18.
16. Prasad S, Wilkinson J, Gatzoulis MA. Sildenafil in primary pulmonary hypertension. N Engl J Med. 2000;343(18):1342.
17. Wilkens H, Guth A, Konig J, Forestier N, Cremers B, Hennen B, et al. Effect of inhaled iloprost plus oral sildenafil in patients with primary pulmonary hypertension. Circulation. 2001; 104(11):1218–22.
18. Lepore JJ, Maroo A, Pereira NL, Ginns LC, Dec GW, Zapol WM, et al. Effect of sildenafil on the acute pulmonary vasodilator response to inhaled nitric oxide in adults with primary pulmonary hypertension. Am J Cardiol. 2002;90(6):677–80.
19. Madden BP, Sheth A, Wilde M, Ong YE. Does Sildenafil produce a sustained benefit in patients with pulmonary hypertension associated with parenchymal lung and cardiac disease? Vascul Pharmacol. 2007;47(2–3):184–8.
20. Sastry BK, Narasimhan C, Reddy NK, Raju BS. Clinical efficacy of sildenafil in primary pulmonary hypertension: a randomized, placebo-controlled, double-blind, crossover study. J Am Coll Cardiol. 2004;43(7):1149–53.
21. Galie N, Ghofrani HA, Torbicki A, Barst RJ, Rubin LJ, Badesch D, et al. Sildenafil citrate therapy for pulmonary arterial hypertension. N Engl J Med. 2005;353(20):2148–57.
22. Pepke-Zaba J, Gilbert C, Collings L, Brown MC. Sildenafil improves health-related quality of life in patients with pulmonary arterial hypertension. Chest. 2008;133(1):183–9.
23. Rubin LJ, Badesch DB, Fleming TR, Galie N, Simonneau G, Ghofrani HA, et al. Long-term treatment with sildenafil citrate in pulmonary arterial hypertension: the SUPER-2 study. Chest. 2011;140(5):1274–83.
24. Galie N, Brundage BH, Ghofrani HA, Oudiz RJ, Simonneau G, Safdar Z, et al. Tadalafil therapy for pulmonary arterial hypertension. Circulation. 2009;119(22):2894–903.
25. Jing ZC, Yu ZX, Shen JY, Wu BX, Xu KF, Zhu XY, et al. Vardenafil in pulmonary arterial hypertension: a randomized, double-blind, placebo-controlled study. Am J Respir Crit Care Med. 2011;183(12):1723–9.
26. Rubin LJ, Mendoza J, Hood M, McGoon M, Barst R, Williams WB, et al. Treatment of primary pulmonary hypertension with continuous intravenous prostacyclin (epoprostenol). Results of a randomized trial. Ann Intern Med. 1990;112(7):485–91.

27. Barst RJ, Rubin LJ, McGoon MD, Caldwell EJ, Long WA, Levy PS. Survival in primary pulmonary hypertension with long-term continuous intravenous prostacyclin. Ann Intern Med. 1994; 121(6):409–15.

28. Barst RJ, Rubin LJ, Long WA, McGoon MD, Rich S, Badesch DB, et al. A comparison of continuous intravenous epoprostenol (prostacyclin) with conventional therapy for primary pulmonary hypertension. N Engl J Med. 1996;334(5):296–301.

29. Higenbottam T, Butt AY, McMahon A, Westerbeck R, Sharples L. Long-term intravenous prostaglandin (epoprostenol or iloprost) for treatment of severe pulmonary hypertension. Heart (British Cardiac Society). 1998;80(2):151–5.

30. Simonneau G, Barst RJ, Galie N, Naeije R, Rich S, Bourge RC, et al. Continuous subcutaneous infusion of treprostinil, a prostacyclin analogue, in patients with pulmonary arterial hypertension: a double-blind, randomized, placebo-controlled trial. Am J Respir Crit Care Med. 2002;165(6):800–4.

31. Tapson VF, Jing ZC, Xu KF, Pan L, Feldman J, Kiely DG, et al. Oral treprostinil for the treatment of pulmonary arterial hypertension in patients receiving background endothelin receptor antagonist and phosphodiesterase type 5 inhibitor therapy (the FREEDOM-C2 study): a randomized controlled trial. Chest. 2013;144(3):952–8.

32. Olschewski H, Simonneau G, Galie N, Higenbottam T, Naeije R, Rubin LJ, et al. Inhaled iloprost for severe pulmonary hypertension. N Engl J Med. 2002;347(5):322–9.

33. Galie N, Humbert M, Vachiery JL, Vizza CD, Kneussl M, Manes A, et al. Effects of beraprost sodium, an oral prostacyclin analogue, in patients with pulmonary arterial hypertension: a randomized, double-blind, placebo-controlled trial. J Am Coll Cardiol. 2002;39(9):1496–502.

34. Barst RJ, McGoon M, McLaughlin V, Tapson V, Rich S, Rubin L, et al. Beraprost therapy for pulmonary arterial hypertension. J Am Coll Cardiol. 2003;41(12):2119–25.

35. Ghofrani HA, Rose F, Schermuly RT, Olschewski H, Wiedemann R, Kreckel A, et al. Oral sildenafil as long-term adjunct therapy to inhaled iloprost in severe pulmonary arterial hypertension. J Am Coll Cardiol. 2003;42(1):158–64.

36. Hoeper MM, Taha N, Bekjarova A, Gatzke R, Spiekerkoetter E. Bosentan treatment in patients with primary pulmonary hypertension receiving nonparenteral prostanoids. Eur Respir J. 2003;22(2):330–4.

37. Hoeper MM, Leuchte H, Halank M, Wilkens H, Meyer FJ, Seyfarth HJ, et al. Combining inhaled iloprost with bosentan in patients with idiopathic pulmonary arterial hypertension. Eur Respir J. 2006;28(4):691–4.

38. McLaughlin VV, Oudiz RJ, Frost A, Tapson VF, Murali S, Channick RN, et al. Randomized study of adding inhaled iloprost to existing bosentan in pulmonary arterial hypertension. Am J Respir Crit Care Med. 2006;174(11):1257–63.

39. Humbert M, Barst RJ, Robbins IM, Channick RN, Galie N, Boonstra A, et al. Combination of bosentan with epoprostenol in pulmonary arterial hypertension: BREATHE-2. Eur Respir J. 2004;24(3):353–9.

40. Simonneau G, Rubin LJ, Galie N, Barst RJ, Fleming TR, Frost AE, et al. Addition of sildenafil to long-term intravenous epoprostenol therapy in patients with pulmonary arterial hypertension: a randomized trial. Ann Intern Med. 2008;149(8):521–30.

41. McLaughlin VV, Benza RL, Rubin LJ, Channick RN, Voswinckel R, Tapson VF, et al. Addition of inhaled treprostinil to oral therapy for pulmonary arterial hypertension: a randomized controlled clinical trial. J Am Coll Cardiol. 2010;55(18):1915–22.

42. Tapson VF, Torres F, Kermeen F, Keogh AM, Allen RP, Frantz RP, et al. Oral treprostinil for the treatment of pulmonary arterial hypertension in patients on background endothelin receptor antagonist and/or phosphodiesterase type 5 inhibitor therapy (the FREEDOM-C study): a randomized controlled trial. Chest. 2012;142(6):1383–90.

43. Sitbon O, Jais X, Savale L, Dauphin C, Natali D, O'Callaghan D, et al. Upfront triple combination therapy of IV epoprostenol with oral bosentan and sildenafil in idiopathic and heritable pulmonary arterial hypertension. Am J Respir Crit Care Med. 2011;183.

44. Sitbon O, Humbert M, Jagot JL, Taravella O, Fartoukh M, Parent F, et al. Inhaled nitric oxide as a screening agent for safely identifying responders to oral calcium-channel blockers in primary pulmonary hypertension. Eur Respir J. 1998;12(2):265–70.

45. Sitbon O, Humbert M, Jais X, Ioos V, Hamid AM, Provencher S, et al. Long-term response to calcium channel blockers in idiopathic pulmonary arterial hypertension. Circulation. 2005;111(23):3105–11.

46. Malhotra R, Hess D, Lewis GD, Bloch KD, Waxman AB, Semigran MJ. Vasoreactivity to inhaled nitric oxide with oxygen predicts long-term survival in pulmonary arterial hypertension. Pulm Circ. 2011;1(2):250–8.

47. Galie N, Hoeper MM, Humbert M, Torbicki A, Vachiery JL, Barbera JA, et al. Guidelines for the diagnosis and treatment of pulmonary hypertension: the Task Force for the Diagnosis and Treatment of Pulmonary Hypertension of the European Society of Cardiology (ESC) and the European Respiratory Society (ERS), endorsed by the International Society of Heart and Lung Transplantation (ISHLT). Eur Heart J. 2009;30(20):2493–537.

48. Galie N, Corris PA, Frost A, Girgis RE, Granton J, Jing ZC, et al. Updated treatment algorithm of pulmonary arterial hypertension. J Am Coll Cardiol. 2013;62(25 Suppl):D60–72.

49. McLaughlin VV, Archer SL, Badesch DB, Barst RJ, Farber HW, Lindner JR, et al. ACCF/AHA 2009 expert consensus document on pulmonary hypertension a report of the American College of Cardiology Foundation Task Force on Expert Consensus Documents and the American Heart Association developed in collaboration with the American College of Chest Physicians; American Thoracic Society, Inc.; and the Pulmonary Hypertension Association. J Am Coll Cardiol. 2009;53(17):1573–619.

50. Johnson SR, Mehta S, Granton JT. Anticoagulation in pulmonary arterial hypertension: a qualitative systematic review. Eur Respir J. 2006;28(5):999–1004.

51. Johnson SR, Granton JT, Mehta S. Thrombotic arteriopathy and anticoagulation in pulmonary hypertension. Chest. 2006; 130(2):545–52.

52. Mathur PN, Powles P, Pugsley SO, McEwan MP, Campbell EJ. Effect of digoxin on right ventricular function in severe chronic airflow obstruction. A controlled clinical trial. Ann Intern Med. 1981;95(3):283–8.

53. Rich S, Seidlitz M, Dodin E, Osimani D, Judd D, Genthner D, et al. The short-term effects of digoxin in patients with right ventricular dysfunction from pulmonary hypertension. Chest. 1998;114(3):787–92.

54. Ghofrani HA, Voswinckel R, Reichenberger F, Weissmann N, Schermuly RT, Seeger W, et al. Hypoxia- and non-hypoxia-related pulmonary hypertension – established and new therapies. Cardiovasc Res. 2006;72(1):30–40.

55. Badesch DB, Raskob GE, Elliott CG, Krichman AM, Farber HW, Frost AE, et al. Pulmonary arterial hypertension: baseline characteristics from the REVEAL Registry. Chest. 2010; 137(2):376–87.

56. Bogaard HJ, Natarajan R, Mizuno S, Abbate A, Chang PJ, Chau VQ, et al. Adrenergic receptor blockade reverses right heart

remodeling and dysfunction in pulmonary hypertensive rats. Am J Respir Crit Care Med. 2010;182(5):652–60.

57. So PP, Davies RA, Chandy G, Stewart D, Beanlands RS, Haddad H, et al. Usefulness of beta-blocker therapy and outcomes in patients with pulmonary arterial hypertension. Am J Cardiol. 2012;109(10):1504–9.

58. Hansdottir S, Groskreutz DJ, Gehlbach BK. WHO's in second? a practical review of World Health Organization Group 2 pulmonary hypertension. Chest. 2013;144(2):638–50.

59. Provencher S, Herve P, Jais X, Lebrec D, Humbert M, Simonneau G, et al. Deleterious effects of beta-blockers on exercise capacity and hemodynamics in patients with portopulmonary hypertension. Gastroenterology. 2006;130(1):120–6.

60. Tongers J, Schwerdtfeger B, Klein G, Kempf T, Schaefer A, Knapp JM, et al. Incidence and clinical relevance of supraventricular tachyarrhythmias in pulmonary hypertension. Am Heart J. 2007;153(1):127–32.

61. MRC. Long term domiciliary oxygen therapy in chronic hypoxic cor pulmonale complicating chronic bronchitis and emphysema. Report of the Medical Research Council Working Party. Lancet. 1981;1(8222):681–6.

62. NOTT. Continuous or nocturnal oxygen therapy in hypoxemic chronic obstructive lung disease: a clinical trial. Nocturnal Oxygen Therapy Trial Group. Ann Intern Med. 1980;93(3):391–8.

63. Weitzenblum E, Sautegeau A, Ehrhart M, Mammosser M, Pelletier A. Long-term oxygen therapy can reverse the progression of pulmonary hypertension in patients with chronic obstructive pulmonary disease. Am Rev Respir Dis. 1985;131(4):493–8.

64. Ashutosh K, Mead G, Dunsky M. Early effects of oxygen administration and prognosis in chronic obstructive pulmonary disease and cor pulmonale. Am Rev Respir Dis. 1983;127(4):399–404.

65. National Clinical Guideline Centre. Chronic obstructive pulmonary disease: management of chronic obstructive pulmonary disease in adults in primary and secondary care. London: National Clinical Guideline Centre; 2010. Available from: http://guidance.nice.org.uk/CG101/Guidance/pdf/English.

66. NICE. National Institute for Health and Care Excellence. Management of chronic obstructive pulmonary disease in adults in primary and secondary care (partial update). Clinical guidelines, CG101 – Issued: June 2010. 2010.

67. Rafanan AL, Golish JA, Dinner DS, Hague LK, Arroliga AC. Nocturnal hypoxemia is common in primary pulmonary hypertension. Chest. 2001;120(3):894–9.
68. Mereles D, Ehlken N, Kreuscher S, Ghofrani S, Hoeper MM, Halank M, et al. Exercise and respiratory training improve exercise capacity and quality of life in patients with severe chronic pulmonary hypertension. Circulation. 2006;114(14):1482–9.
69. Grunig E, Lichtblau M, Ehlken N, Ghofrani HA, Reichenberger F, Staehler G, et al. Safety and efficacy of exercise training in various forms of pulmonary hypertension. Eur Respir J. 2012; 40(1):84–92.
70. Chan L, Chin LM, Kennedy M, Woolstenhulme JG, Nathan SD, Weinstein AA, et al. Benefits of intensive treadmill exercise training on cardiorespiratory function and quality of life in patients with pulmonary hypertension. Chest. 2013;143(2): 333–43.
71. Weinstein AA, Chin LM, Keyser RE, Kennedy M, Nathan SD, Woolstenhulme JG, et al. Effect of aerobic exercise training on fatigue and physical activity in patients with pulmonary arterial hypertension. Respir Med. 2013;107(5):778–84.
72. Souza R, Humbert M, Sztrymf B, Jais X, Yaici A, Le Pavec J, et al. Pulmonary arterial hypertension associated with fenfluramine exposure: report of 109 cases. Eur Respir J. 2008;31(2):343–8.
73. Montani D, Savale L, Natali D, Jais X, Herve P, Garcia G, et al. Long-term response to calcium-channel blockers in non-idiopathic pulmonary arterial hypertension. Eur Heart J. 2010;31(15):1898–907.
74. Denton CP, Pope JE, Peter HH, Gabrielli A, Boonstra A, van den Hoogen FH, et al. Long-term effects of bosentan on quality of life, survival, safety and tolerability in pulmonary arterial hypertension related to connective tissue diseases. Ann Rheum Dis. 2008;67(9):1222–8.
75. Badesch DB, Tapson VF, McGoon MD, Brundage BH, Rubin LJ, Wigley FM, et al. Continuous intravenous epoprostenol for pulmonary hypertension due to the scleroderma spectrum of disease. A randomized, controlled trial. Ann Intern Med. 2000;132(6):425–34.
76. Jais X, Launay D, Yaici A, Le Pavec J, Tcherakian C, Sitbon O, et al. Immunosuppressive therapy in lupus- and mixed connective tissue disease-associated pulmonary arterial hypertension: a retrospective analysis of twenty-three cases. Arthritis Rheum. 2008;58(2):521–31.
77. Overbeek MJ, Vonk MC, Boonstra A, Voskuyl AE, Vonk-Noordegraaf A, Smit EF, et al. Pulmonary arterial hypertension

in limited cutaneous systemic sclerosis: a distinctive vasculopathy. Eur Respir J. 2009;34(2):371–9.

78. Gingo MR, Morris A. Pathogenesis of HIV and the lung. Curr HIV/AIDS Rep. 2013;10(1):42–50.

79. Zuber JP, Calmy A, Evison JM, Hasse B, Schiffer V, Wagels T, et al. Pulmonary arterial hypertension related to HIV infection: improved hemodynamics and survival associated with antiretroviral therapy. Clin Infect Dis Off Publ Infect Dis Soc Am. 2004;38(8):1178–85.

80. Opravil M, Pechere M, Speich R, Joller-Jemelka HI, Jenni R, Russi EW, et al. HIV-associated primary pulmonary hypertension. A case control study. Swiss HIV Cohort Study. Am J Respir Crit Care Med. 1997;155(3):990–5.

81. Degano B, Guillaume M, Savale L, Montani D, Jais X, Yaici A, et al. HIV-associated pulmonary arterial hypertension: survival and prognostic factors in the modern therapeutic era. AIDS (London, England). 2010;24(1):67–75.

82. Aschmann YZ, Kummer O, Linka A, Wenk M, Azzola A, Bodmer M, et al. Pharmacokinetics and pharmacodynamics of sildenafil in a patient treated with human immunodeficiency virus protease inhibitors. Ther Drug Monit. 2008;30(1):130–4.

83. Chinello P, Cicalini S, Pichini S, Pacifici R, Tempestilli M, Petrosillo N. Sildenafil plasma concentrations in two HIV patients with pulmonary hypertension treated with ritonavir-boosted protease inhibitors. Curr HIV Res. 2012;10(2):162–4.

84. McRae MP, Lowe CM, Tian X, Bourdet DL, Ho RH, Leake BF, et al. Ritonavir, saquinavir, and efavirenz, but not nevirapine, inhibit bile acid transport in human and rat hepatocytes. J Pharmacol Exp Ther. 2006;318(3):1068–75.

85. Dingemanse J, van Giersbergen PL, Patat A, Nilsson PN. Mutual pharmacokinetic interactions between bosentan and lopinavir/ritonavir in healthy participants. Antivir Ther. 2010;15(2):157–63.

86. Panel on Antiretroviral Guidelines for Adults and Adolescents. Guidelines for the use of antiretroviral agents in HIV-infected adults and adolescents. Department of Health and Human Services. Federal register October 2011. p. 1–167. Available from: http://www.aidsinfo.nih.gov/ContentFiles/AdultandAdolescentGL.pdf.

87. Bristol-Myers Squibb Canada. Reytaz (atazanavir) Product monograph. Montreal; 2011.

88. Sitbon O, Gressin V, Speich R, Macdonald PS, Opravil M, Cooper DA, et al. Bosentan for the treatment of human immunodeficiency virus-associated pulmonary arterial hypertension. Am J Respir Crit Care Med. 2004;170(11):1212–7.

89. Barbaro G, Lucchini A, Pellicelli AM, Grisorio B, Giancaspro G, Barbarini G. Highly active antiretroviral therapy compared with HAART and bosentan in combination in patients with HIV-associated pulmonary hypertension. Heart (British Cardiac Society). 2006;92(8):1164–6.

90. Nunes H, Humbert M, Sitbon O, Morse JH, Deng Z, Knowles JA, et al. Prognostic factors for survival in human immunodeficiency virus-associated pulmonary arterial hypertension. Am J Respir Crit Care Med. 2003;167(10):1433–9.

91. Aguilar RV, Farber HW. Epoprostenol (prostacyclin) therapy in HIV-associated pulmonary hypertension. Am J Respir Crit Care Med. 2000;162(5):1846–50.

92. Petitpretz P, Brenot F, Azarian R, Parent F, Rain B, Herve P, et al. Pulmonary hypertension in patients with human immunodeficiency virus infection. Comparison with primary pulmonary hypertension. Circulation. 1994;89(6):2722–7.

93. Cea-Calvo L, Escribano Subias P, Tello de Menesses R, Lazaro Salvador M, Gomez Sanchez MA, Delgado Jimenez JF, et al. Treatment of HIV-associated pulmonary hypertension with treprostinil. Rev Esp Cardiol. 2003;56(4):421–5.

94. Ghofrani HA, Friese G, Discher T, Olschewski H, Schermuly RT, Weissmann N, et al. Inhaled iloprost is a potent acute pulmonary vasodilator in HIV-related severe pulmonary hypertension. Eur Respir J. 2004;23(2):321–6.

95. Hadengue A, Benhayoun MK, Lebrec D, Benhamou JP. Pulmonary hypertension complicating portal hypertension: prevalence and relation to splanchnic hemodynamics. Gastroenterology. 1991;100(2):520–8.

96. Ramsay MA, Simpson BR, Nguyen AT, Ramsay KJ, East C, Klintmalm GB. Severe pulmonary hypertension in liver transplant candidates. Liver Transpl Surg Off Publ Am Assoc Study Liver Dis Int Liver Transpl Soc. 1997;3(5):494–500.

97. Pellicelli AM, Barbaro G, Puoti C, Guarascio P, Lusi EA, Bellis L, et al. Plasma cytokines and portopulmonary hypertension in patients with cirrhosis waiting for orthotopic liver transplantation. Angiology. 2010;61(8):802–6.

98. Hoeper MM, Halank M, Marx C, Hoeffken G, Seyfarth HJ, Schauer J, et al. Bosentan therapy for portopulmonary hypertension. Eur Respir J. 2005;25(3):502–8.

99. Kuo PC, Johnson LB, Plotkin JS, Howell CD, Bartlett ST, Rubin LJ. Continuous intravenous infusion of epoprostenol for the treatment of portopulmonary hypertension. Transplantation. 1997;63(4):604–6.

100. Reichenberger F, Voswinckel R, Steveling E, Enke B, Kreckel A, Olschewski H, et al. Sildenafil treatment for portopulmonary hypertension. Eur Respir J. 2006;28(3):563–7.
101. Findlay JY, Plevak DJ, Krowka MJ, Sack EM, Porayko MK. Progressive splenomegaly after epoprostenol therapy in portopulmonary hypertension. Liver Transpl Surg Off Publ Am Assoc Study Liver Dis Int Liver Transpl Soc. 1999;5(5):362–5.
102. Savale L, Magnier R, Le Pavec J, Jais X, Montani D, O'Callaghan DS, et al. Efficacy, safety and pharmacokinetics of bosentan in portopulmonary hypertension. Eur Respir J. 2013;41(1):96–103.
103. Schott R, Chaouat A, Launoy A, Pottecher T, Weitzenblum E. Improvement of pulmonary hypertension after liver transplantation. Chest. 1999;115(6):1748–9.
104. Beghetti M, Galie N. Eisenmenger syndrome a clinical perspective in a new therapeutic era of pulmonary arterial hypertension. J Am Coll Cardiol. 2009;53(9):733–40.
105. Galie N, Beghetti M, Gatzoulis MA, Granton J, Berger RM, Lauer A, et al. Bosentan therapy in patients with Eisenmenger syndrome: a multicenter, double-blind, randomized, placebo-controlled study. Circulation. 2006;114(1):48–54.
106. Chau EM, Fan KY, Chow WH. Effects of chronic sildenafil in patients with Eisenmenger syndrome versus idiopathic pulmonary arterial hypertension. Int J Cardiol. 2007;120(3):301–5.
107. Beciani E, Palazzini M, Bulatovic I, Mazzanti G, Gotti E, Marinelli A, et al. Effects of sildenafil treatment in patients with pulmonary hypertension associated with congenital cardiac shunts. Am J Respir Crit Care Med. 2010;181.
108. Dimopoulos K, Inuzuka R, Goletto S, Giannakoulas G, Swan L, Wort SJ, et al. Improved survival among patients with Eisenmenger syndrome receiving advanced therapy for pulmonary arterial hypertension. Circulation. 2010;121(1):20–5.
109. Sandoval J, Aguirre JS, Pulido T, Martinez-Guerra ML, Santos E, Alvarado P, et al. Nocturnal oxygen therapy in patients with the Eisenmenger syndrome. Am J Respir Crit Care Med. 2001;164(9):1682–7.
110. Lapa M, Dias B, Jardim C, Fernandes CJ, Dourado PM, Figueiredo M, et al. Cardiopulmonary manifestations of hepatosplenic schistosomiasis. Circulation. 2009;119(11):1518–23.
111. Correa Rde A, Moreira MV, Saraiva JM, Mancuzo EV, Silva LC, Lambertucci JR. Treatment of schistosomiasis-associated pulmonary hypertension. Jornal brasileiro de pneumologia publicacao oficial da Sociedade Brasileira de Pneumologia e Tisilogia. 2011;37(2):272–6.

112. Graham BB, Bandeira AP, Morrell NW, Butrous G, Tuder RM. Schistosomiasis-associated pulmonary hypertension: pulmonary vascular disease: the global perspective. Chest. 2010; 137(6 Suppl):20s–9.

113. Fernandes CJ, Dias BA, Jardim CV, Hovnanian A, Hoette S, Morinaga LK, et al. The role of target therapies in schistosomiasis-associated pulmonary arterial hypertension. Chest. 2012;141(4): 923–8.

114. Palmer SM, Robinson LJ, Wang A, Gossage JR, Bashore T, Tapson VF. Massive pulmonary edema and death after prostacyclin infusion in a patient with pulmonary veno-occlusive disease. Chest. 1998;113(1):237–40.

115. Okumura H, Nagaya N, Kyotani S, Sakamaki F, Nakanishi N, Fukuhara S, et al. Effects of continuous IV prostacyclin in a patient with pulmonary veno-occlusive disease. Chest. 2002;122(3):1096–8.

116. Montani D, Jais X, Price LC, Achouh L, Degano B, Mercier O, et al. Cautious epoprostenol therapy is a safe bridge to lung transplantation in pulmonary veno-occlusive disease. Eur Respir J. 2009;34(6):1348–56.

117. Sanderson JE, Spiro SG, Hendry AT, Turner-Warwick M. A case of pulmonary veno-occlusive disease respondong to treatment with azathioprine. Thorax. 1977;32(2):140–8.

118. Califf RM, Adams KF, McKenna WJ, Gheorghiade M, Uretsky BF, McNulty SE, et al. A randomized controlled trial of epoprostenol therapy for severe congestive heart failure: The Flolan International Randomized Survival Trial (FIRST). Am Heart J. 1997;134(1):44–54.

119. Ferguson JJ. Meeting highlights: highlights of the 51st annual scientific sessions of the American College of Cardiology. Atlanta, Georgia, USA. March 17–20, 2002. Circulation. 2002;106(7):E24–30.

120. Guazzi M, Vicenzi M, Arena R, Guazzi MD. Pulmonary hypertension in heart failure with preserved ejection fraction: a target of phosphodiesterase-5 inhibition in a 1-year study. Circulation. 2011;124(2):164–74.

121. Lewis GD, Shah R, Shahzad K, Camuso JM, Pappagianopoulos PP, Hung J, et al. Sildenafil improves exercise capacity and quality of life in patients with systolic heart failure and secondary pulmonary hypertension. Circulation. 2007;116(14):1555–62.

122. Madden BP, Allenby M, Loke TK, Sheth A. A potential role for sildenafil in the management of pulmonary hypertension in

patients with parenchymal lung disease. Vascul Pharmacol. 2006;44(5):372–6.

123. Blanco I, Gimeno E, Munoz PA, Pizarro S, Gistau C, Rodriguez-Roisin R, et al. Hemodynamic and gas exchange effects of sildenafil in patients with chronic obstructive pulmonary disease and pulmonary hypertension. Am J Respir Crit Care Med. 2010;181(3):270–8.

124. Rao RS, Singh S, Sharma BB, Agarwal VV, Singh V. Sildenafil improves six-minute walk distance in chronic obstructive pulmonary disease: a randomised, double-blind, placebo-controlled trial. Indian J Chest Dis Allied Sci. 2011;53(2):81–5.

125. Shujaat A, Bajwa AA, Cury JD. Pulmonary hypertension secondary to COPD. Pulm Med. 2012;2012:203952.

126. Lee TM, Chen CC, Shen HN, Chang NC. Effects of pravastatin on functional capacity in patients with chronic obstructive pulmonary disease and pulmonary hypertension. Clin Sci (London, England: 1979). 2009;116(6):497–505.

127. Ghofrani HA, Wiedemann R, Rose F, Schermuly RT, Olschewski H, Weissmann N, et al. Sildenafil for treatment of lung fibrosis and pulmonary hypertension: a randomised controlled trial. Lancet. 2002;360(9337):895–900.

128. Olschewski H, Ghofrani HA, Walmrath D, Schermuly R, Temmesfeld-Wollbruck B, Grimminger F, et al. Inhaled prostacyclin and iloprost in severe pulmonary hypertension secondary to lung fibrosis. Am J Respir Crit Care Med. 1999;160(2):600–7.

129. King Jr TE, Behr J, Brown KK, du Bois RM, Lancaster L, de Andrade JA, et al. BUILD-1: a randomized placebo-controlled trial of bosentan in idiopathic pulmonary fibrosis. Am J Respir Crit Care Med. 2008;177(1):75–81.

130. King Jr TE, Brown KK, Raghu G, du Bois RM, Lynch DA, Martinez F, et al. BUILD-3: a randomized, controlled trial of bosentan in idiopathic pulmonary fibrosis. Am J Respir Crit Care Med. 2011;184(1):92–9.

131. Seibold JR, Denton CP, Furst DE, Guillevin L, Rubin LJ, Wells A, et al. Randomized, prospective, placebo-controlled trial of bosentan in interstitial lung disease secondary to systemic sclerosis. Arthritis Rheum. 2010;62(7):2101–8.

132. Arias MA, Garcia-Rio F, Alonso-Fernandez A, Martinez I, Villamor J. Pulmonary hypertension in obstructive sleep apnoea: effects of continuous positive airway pressure: a randomized, controlled cross-over study. Eur Heart J. 2006;27(9):1106–13.

133. Sugerman HJ, Baron PL, Fairman RP, Evans CR, Vetrovec GW. Hemodynamic dysfunction in obesity hypoventilation syndrome and the effects of treatment with surgically induced weight loss. Ann Surg. 1988;207(5):604–13.

134. Fedullo P, Kerr KM, Kim NH, Auger WR. Chronic thromboembolic pulmonary hypertension. Am J Respir Crit Care Med. 2011;183(12):1605–13.

135. Jais X, D'Armini AM, Jansa P, Torbicki A, Delcroix M, Ghofrani HA, et al. Bosentan for treatment of inoperable chronic thromboembolic pulmonary hypertension: BENEFiT (Bosentan Effects in iNopErable Forms of chronIc Thromboembolic pulmonary hypertension), a randomized, placebo-controlled trial. J Am Coll Cardiol. 2008;52(25):2127–34.

136. Becattini C, Manina G, Busti C, Gennarini S, Agnelli G. Bosentan for chronic thromboembolic pulmonary hypertension: findings from a systematic review and meta-analysis. Thromb Res. 2010;126(1):e51–6.

137. Sheth A, Park JE, Ong YE, Ho TB, Madden BP. Early haemodynamic benefit of sildenafil in patients with coexisting chronic thromboembolic pulmonary hypertension and left ventricular dysfunction. Vascul Pharmacol. 2005;42(2):41–5.

138. Suntharalingam J, Treacy CM, Doughty NJ, Goldsmith K, Soon E, Toshner MR, et al. Long-term use of sildenafil in inoperable chronic thromboembolic pulmonary hypertension. Chest. 2008;134(2):229–36.

139. Cabrol S, Souza R, Jais X, Fadel E, Ali RH, Humbert M, et al. Intravenous epoprostenol in inoperable chronic thromboembolic pulmonary hypertension. J Heart Lung Transpl Off Publ Int Soc Heart Transpl. 2007;26(4):357–62.

140. Skoro-Sajer N, Bonderman D, Wiesbauer F, Harja E, Jakowitsch J, Klepetko W, et al. Treprostinil for severe inoperable chronic thromboembolic pulmonary hypertension. J Thromb Haemost JTH. 2007;5(3):483–9.

141. Nagaya N, Sasaki N, Ando M, Ogino H, Sakamaki F, Kyotani S, et al. Prostacyclin therapy before pulmonary thromboendarterectomy in patients with chronic thromboembolic pulmonary hypertension. Chest. 2003;123(2):338–43.

142. Jensen KW, Kerr KM, Fedullo PF, Kim NH, Test VJ, Ben-Yehuda O, et al. Pulmonary hypertensive medical therapy in chronic thromboembolic pulmonary hypertension before pulmonary thromboendarterectomy. Circulation. 2009;120(13):1248–54.

143. Condliffe R, Kiely DG, Gibbs JS, Corris PA, Peacock AJ, Jenkins DP, et al. Improved outcomes in medically and surgically treated chronic thromboembolic pulmonary hypertension. Am J Respir Crit Care Med. 2008;177(10):1122–7.

144. Simonneau G, Gatzoulis MA, Adatia I, Celermajer D, Denton C, Ghofrani A, et al. Updated clinical classification of pulmonary hypertension. J Am Coll Cardiol. 2013;62(25 Suppl):D34–41.

145. Miller AC, Gladwin MT. Pulmonary complications of sickle cell disease. Am J Respir Crit Care Med. 2012;185(11):1154–65.

146. Morris CR, Morris Jr SM, Hagar W, Van Warmerdam J, Claster S, Kepka-Lenhart D, et al. Arginine therapy: a new treatment for pulmonary hypertension in sickle cell disease? Am J Respir Crit Care Med. 2003;168(1):63–9.

147. Nunes H, Humbert M, Capron F, Brauner M, Sitbon O, Battesti JP, et al. Pulmonary hypertension associated with sarcoidosis: mechanisms, haemodynamics and prognosis. Thorax. 2006;61(1):68–74.

148. Corte TJ, Wells AU, Nicholson AG, Hansell DM, Wort SJ. Pulmonary hypertension in sarcoidosis: a review. Respirology (Carlton, Vic). 2011;16(1):69–77.

149. Fisher KA, Serlin DM, Wilson KC, Walter RE, Berman JS, Farber HW. Sarcoidosis-associated pulmonary hypertension: outcome with long-term epoprostenol treatment. Chest. 2006;130(5):1481–8.

150. Milman N, Burton CM, Iversen M, Videbaek R, Jensen CV, Carlsen J. Pulmonary hypertension in end-stage pulmonary sarcoidosis: therapeutic effect of sildenafil? J Heart Lung Transpl Off Publ Int Soc Heart Transpl. 2008;27(3):329–34.

151. Baughman RP, Culver DA, Cordova FC, Padilla M, Gibson KF, Lower EE, et al. Bosentan for sarcoidosis associated pulmonary hypertension: a double-blind placebo controlled randomized trial. Chest. 2014;145(4):810–7.

152. Barnett CF, Bonura EJ, Nathan SD, Ahmad S, Shlobin OA, Osei K, et al. Treatment of sarcoidosis-associated pulmonary hypertension. A two-center experience. Chest. 2009;135(6):1455–61.

153. Shrikrishna D, Coker RK. Managing passengers with stable respiratory disease planning air travel: British Thoracic Society recommendations. Thorax. 2011;66(9):831–3.

154. Madden BP. Pulmonary hypertension and pregnancy. Int J Obstet Anesth. 2009;18(2):156–64.

155. Clapp 3rd JF, Capeless E. Cardiovascular function before, during, and after the first and subsequent pregnancies. Am J Cardiol. 1997;80(11):1469–73.

156. Daliento L, Somerville J, Presbitero P, Menti L, Brach-Prever S, Rizzoli G, et al. Eisenmenger syndrome. Factors relating to deterioration and death. Eur Heart J. 1998;19(12):1845–55.
157. Kiely DG, Condliffe R, Webster V, Mills GH, Wrench I, Gandhi SV, et al. Improved survival in pregnancy and pulmonary hypertension using a multiprofessional approach. BJOG. 2010;117(5):565–74.
158. Goland S, Tsai F, Habib M, Janmohamed M, Goodwin TM, Elkayam U. Favorable outcome of pregnancy with an elective use of epoprostenol and sildenafil in women with severe pulmonary hypertension. Cardiology. 2010;115(3):205–8.
159. Gurakan B, Kayiran P, Ozturk N, Kayiran SM, Dindar A. Therapeutic combination of sildenafil and iloprost in a preterm neonate with pulmonary hypertension. Pediatr Pulmonol. 2011;46(6):617–20.
160. Villanueva-Garcia D, Mota-Rojas D, Hernandez-Gonzalez R, Sanchez-Aparicio P, Alonso-Spilsbury M, Trujillo-Ortega ME, et al. A systematic review of experimental and clinical studies of sildenafil citrate for intrauterine growth restriction and preterm labour. J Obstet Gynaecol J Institute Obstet Gynaecol. 2007;27(3):255–9.
161. Lacassie HJ, Germain AM, Valdes G, Fernandez MS, Allamand F, Lopez H. Management of Eisenmenger syndrome in pregnancy with sildenafil and L-arginine. Obstet Gynecol. 2004;103(5 Pt 2):1118–20.
162. Iacovidou N, Syggelou A, Fanos V, Xanthos T. The use of sildenafil in the treatment of persistent pulmonary hypertension of the newborn: a review of the literature. Curr Pharm Des. 2012;18(21):3034–45.
163. Elliot CA, Stewart P, Webster VJ, Mills GH, Hutchinson SP, Howarth ES, et al. The use of iloprost in early pregnancy in patients with pulmonary arterial hypertension. Eur Respir J. 2005;26(1):168–73.
164. Cotrim SC, Loureiro MJ, Avillez T, Simoes O, Cordeiro P, Almeida S, et al. Three cases of pregnancy in patients with severe pulmonary arterial hypertension: experience of a single unit. Rev Port Cardiol. 2010;29(1):95–103.
165. Badalian SS, Silverman RK, Aubry RH, Longo J. Twin pregnancy in a woman on long-term epoprostenol therapy for primary pulmonary hypertension. A case report. J Reprod Med. 2000;45(2):149–52.
166. Avdalovic M, Sandrock C, Hoso A, Allen R, Albertson TE. Epoprostenol in pregnant patients with secondary

pulmonary hypertension: two case reports and a review of the literature. Treat Respir Med. 2004;3(1):29–34.

167. Kiss H, Egarter C, Asseryanis E, Putz D, Kneussl M. Primary pulmonary hypertension in pregnancy: a case report. Am J Obstet Gynecol. 1995;172(3):1052–4.

168. Magee LA, Schick B, Donnenfeld AE, Sage SR, Conover B, Cook L, et al. The safety of calcium channel blockers in human pregnancy: a prospective, multicenter cohort study. Am J Obstet Gynecol. 1996;174(3):823–8.

169. Budts W, Van Pelt N, Gillyns H, Gewillig M, Van De Werf F, Janssens S. Residual pulmonary vasoreactivity to inhaled nitric oxide in patients with severe obstructive pulmonary hypertension and Eisenmenger syndrome. Heart (British Cardiac Society). 2001;86(5):553–8.

170. Leuchte HH, Schwaiblmair M, Baumgartner RA, Neurohr CF, Kolbe T, Behr J. Hemodynamic response to sildenafil, nitric oxide, and iloprost in primary pulmonary hypertension. Chest. 2004;125(2):580–6.

171. Ulrich S, Fischler M, Speich R, Popov V, Maggiorini M. Chronic thromboembolic and pulmonary arterial hypertension share acute vasoreactivity properties. Chest. 2006;130(3):841–6.

172. Goodwin TM, Gherman RB, Hameed A, Elkayam U. Favorable response of Eisenmenger syndrome to inhaled nitric oxide during pregnancy. Am J Obstet Gynecol. 1999;180(1 Pt 1):64–7.

173. Lam GK, Stafford RE, Thorp J, Moise Jr KJ, Cairns BA. Inhaled nitric oxide for primary pulmonary hypertension in pregnancy. Obstet Gynecol. 2001;98(5 Pt 2):895–8.

174. Madsen KM, Neerhof MG, Wessale JL, Thaete LG. Influence of ET(B) receptor antagonism on pregnancy outcome in rats. J Soc Gynecol Investig. 2001;8(4):239–44.

175. Bedard E, Dimopoulos K, Gatzoulis MA. Has there been any progress made on pregnancy outcomes among women with pulmonary arterial hypertension? Eur Heart J. 2009;30(3): 256–65.

176. Weiss BM, Zemp L, Seifert B, Hess OM. Outcome of pulmonary vascular disease in pregnancy: a systematic overview from 1978 through 1996. J Am Coll Cardiol. 1998;31(7):1650–7.

177. Martinez MV, Rutherford JD. Pulmonary hypertension in pregnancy. Cardiol Rev. 2013;21(4):167–73.

178. Galie N, Palazzini M, Manes A. Pulmonary arterial hypertension: from the kingdom of the near-dead to multiple clinical trial meta-analyses. Eur Heart J. 2010;31(17):2080–6.

179. Ghofrani HA, Galie N, Grimminger F, Grunig E, Humbert M, Jing ZC, et al. Riociguat for the treatment of pulmonary arterial hypertension. N Engl J Med. 2013;369(4):330–40.

180. Ghofrani HA, D'Armini AM, Grimminger F, Hoeper MM, Jansa P, Kim NH, et al. Riociguat for the treatment of chronic thromboembolic pulmonary hypertension. N Engl J Med. 2013;369(4):319–29.

181. Bonderman D, Ghio S, Felix SB, Ghofrani HA, Michelakis E, Mitrovic V, et al. Riociguat for patients with pulmonary hypertension caused by systolic left ventricular dysfunction: a phase IIb double-blind, randomized, placebo-controlled, dose-ranging hemodynamic study. Circulation. 2013;128(5):502–11.

182. Hoeper MM, Halank M, Wilkens H, Gunther A, Weimann G, Gebert I, et al. Riociguat for interstitial lung disease and pulmonary hypertension: a pilot trial. Eur Respir J. 2013;41(4):853–60.

183. Ghofrani HA, Staehler G, Gruenig E, Halank M, Mitrovic V, Unger S, et al. The Effect of the soluble guanylate cyclase stimulator riociguat on hemodynamics in patients with pulmonary hypertension due to chronic obstructive pulmonary disease. Am J Respir Crit Care Med. 2011;183.

184. Simonneau G, Torbicki A, Hoeper MM, Delcroix M, Karlocai K, Galie N, et al. Selexipag: an oral, selective prostacyclin receptor agonist for the treatment of pulmonary arterial hypertension. Eur Respir J. 2012;40(4):874–80.

185. Hoeper MM, Barst RJ, Bourge RC, Feldman J, Frost AE, Galie N, et al. Imatinib mesylate as add-on therapy for pulmonary arterial hypertension: results of the randomized IMPRES study. Circulation. 2013;127(10):1128–38.

186. Gomberg-Maitland M, Maitland ML, Barst RJ, Sugeng L, Coslet S, Perrino TJ, et al. A dosing/cross-development study of the multikinase inhibitor sorafenib in patients with pulmonary arterial hypertension. Clin Pharmacol Ther. 2010;87(3):303–10.

187. Galie N, Badesch D, Fleming T, Simonneau G, Rubin L, Ewert R, et al. Effects of inhaled aviptadil (vasoactive intestinal peptide) in patients with pulmonary arterial hypertension (PAH): results from a phase II study. Eur Heart J. 2010;31:22.

188. Nagaya N, Kyotani S, Uematsu M, Ueno K, Oya H, Nakanishi N, et al. Effects of adrenomedullin inhalation on hemodynamics and exercise capacity in patients with idiopathic pulmonary arterial hypertension. Circulation. 2004;109(3):351–6.

189. Fujita H, Fukumoto Y, Saji K, Sugimura K, Demachi J, Nawata J, et al. Acute vasodilator effects of inhaled fasudil, a specific

Rho-kinase inhibitor, in patients with pulmonary arterial hypertension. Heart Vessels. 2010;25(2):144–9.

190. Wilkins MR, Ali O, Bradlow W, Wharton J, Taegtmeyer A, Rhodes CJ, et al. Simvastatin as a treatment for pulmonary hypertension trial. Am J Respir Crit Care Med. 2010;181(10):1106–13.

191. Kawut SM, Bagiella E, Lederer DJ, Shimbo D, Horn EM, Roberts KE, et al. Randomized clinical trial of aspirin and simvastatin for pulmonary arterial hypertension: ASA-STAT. Circulation. 2011;123(25):2985–93.

192. Channick RN, Newhart JW, Johnson FW, Williams PJ, Auger WR, Fedullo PF, et al. Pulsed delivery of inhaled nitric oxide to patients with primary pulmonary hypertension: an ambulatory delivery system and initial clinical tests. Chest. 1996;109(6):1545–9.

193. Snell GI, Salamonsen RF, Bergin P, Esmore DS, Khan S, Williams TJ. Inhaled nitric oxide used as a bridge to heart-lung transplantation in a patient with end-stage pulmonary hypertension. Am J Respir Crit Care Med. 1995;151(4):1263–6.

194. Waxman AB, Lawler L, Cornett G. Cicletanine for the treatment of pulmonary arterial hypertension. Arch Intern Med. 2008;168(19):2164–6.

195. Guignabert C, Tu L, Izikki M, Dewachter L, Zadigue P, Humbert M, et al. Dichloroacetate treatment partially regresses established pulmonary hypertension in mice with SM22alpha-targeted overexpression of the serotonin transporter. FASEB J Off Publ Federation Am Soc Exp Biol. 2009;23(12):4135–47.

196. Seferian A, Simonneau G. Therapies for pulmonary arterial hypertension: where are we today, where do we go tomorrow? Eur Respir Rev Off J Eur Respir Soc. 2013;22(129):217–26.

197. Diller GP, Thum T, Wilkins MR, Wharton J. Endothelial progenitor cells in pulmonary arterial hypertension. Trends Cardiovasc Med. 2010;20(1):22–9.

198. Wang XX, Zhang FR, Shang YP, Zhu JH, Xie XD, Tao QM, et al. Transplantation of autologous endothelial progenitor cells may be beneficial in patients with idiopathic pulmonary arterial hypertension: a pilot randomized controlled trial. J Am Coll Cardiol. 2007;49(14):1566–71.

199. Reynolds AM, Holmes MD, Danilov SM, Reynolds PN. Targeted gene delivery of BMPR2 attenuates pulmonary hypertension. Eur Respir J. 2012;39(2):329–43.

Chapter 4
The Role of Surgery in Pulmonary Hypertension

Caroline Patterson

Introduction

The past three decades have seen parallel advancement in medical and surgical treatment options for pulmonary hypertension. The greatest impact on survival has been achieved through innovations in pulmonary vasodilator use (principally, the discovery of eproprostenol) and transplantation. Surgical intervention is typically considered in patients whose disease is refractory or progresses despite maximal medical therapy. In chronic thromboembolic pulmonary hypertension, where surgery is the only definitive treatment, surgery is considered as soon as the diagnosis is confirmed. All surgery for pulmonary hypertension should be performed in centres with experience and expertise in these techniques.

This chapter will consider the indications, peri-operative management and outcome of pulmonary thromboendarterectomy, atrial septostomy and transplantation as well as the developing roles for right ventricular assist devices and extracorporeal membrane oxygenation in patients with pulmonary hypertension.

C. Patterson
Department of Respiratory Medicine, St. George's Hospital, London, UK
e-mail: carolinemariepatterson@nhs.net

B. Madden (ed.), *Treatment of Pulmonary Hypertension*,
Current Cardiovascular Therapy,
DOI 10.1007/978-3-319-13581-6_4,
© Springer International Publishing Switzerland 2015

147

Pulmonary Thromboendarterectomy

Pulmonary thromboendarterectomy (PTE) is the procedure by which organised and incorporated fibrous obstructive tissue is removed from the pulmonary arterial tree. PTE is the only recognised cure for chronic thromboembolic pulmonary hypertension (CTEPH) and should be considered for all patients with the condition. Nevertheless, a significant proportion of patients with CTEPH are unsuitable for PTE and up to 35 % of patients undergoing surgery have persistent pulmonary hypertension following the procedure [1, 2]. Thus, medical management also has a role to stabilise and improve pulmonary haemodynamics following surgical assessment.

Persistent pulmonary hypertension is more prevalent with distal thromboembolic disease, presumably associated with co-existent small-vessel arteriopathy. Early surgical intervention is believed to reduce the risk of progression to irreversible (secondary) vasculopathy; however, some patients with severe microvascular disease may have primary vasculopathy with secondary thrombosis [3].

Patient Selection

At present, there is no standardised pre-operative classification system for CTEPH to define patients suitable for surgical intervention, although proposals have been made [3]. There is evidence of variability between centres and countries in the selection of patients for PTE. Data from the international CTEPH registry suggests at time of diagnosis, around 63 % of patients are considered operable and around 57 % (range 12–61 % across countries) ultimately undergo surgery. Operable patients are younger but have comparable disease severity (measured by NYHA functional class) to inoperable patients. Low-volume surgical centres, historically performing less than 10 PTEs per year, report higher percentages of inoperable patients, suggesting centre expertise may influence the decision to operate [4].

Operability has traditionally been determined by the degree of proximal thromboembolic disease accessible to surgery, the degree of microvascular disease (suggested by a high peripheral vascular resistance in the absence of substantial chronic thromboembolic disease on angiography), an acceptable surgical risk and patient consent for the procedure. CTEPH registry data indicates the main causes of inoperability are surgically inaccessible disease, imbalances between increased PVR and the amount of accessible disease, PVR greater than 1,500 dyn/s/cm^{-5} (equivalent to 18.75 Wood Units (WU)), age and comorbidity [4].

Pre-operative Assessment

Non-invasive imaging techniques including echocardiography, ventilation-perfusion scanning and computed tomography angiography are widely used in the diagnostic workup of patients with suspected CTEPH. MRI has an increasing role in the morphological, anatomical and functional assessment of cardiopulmonary circulation. Right heart catheterisation with pulmonary angiography remains the gold standard for the confirmation of CTEPH and the assessment of operability [5].

Pulmonary angiography facilitates evaluation of thrombus distribution within the pulmonary vasculature. Patients with thrombus originating in the main, lobar and segmental arteries are generally characterised as having proximal disease, which is more surgically accessible. In the future, pulmonary intravascular ultrasound may become more widely used to determine suitability for PTE. Pulmonary artery occlusion waveform analysis is being used in the research setting but is yet to be adopted in routine clinical practice.

Once the thrombus distribution has been determined, the clinician must decide whether the proportion of proximal disease is sufficient that thromboendarterectomy will decrease pulmonary vascular resistance. Nevertheless, proximal disease is not the sole determinant of whether PTE will be successful and preoperative assessment of the degree and

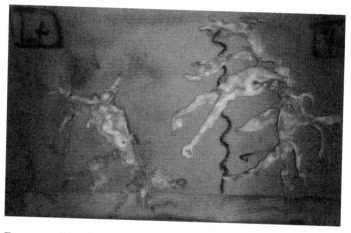

Figure 4.1 Material removed at pulmonary thromboendarterectomy, courtesy of Dr J Haney, Duke University Medical Center

contribution of microvascular disease is essential. Assessment is largely subjective, based on haemodynamic and radiographic findings, but PVR is a useful objective measure.

Surgical Technique

Although supportive evidence is limited, it is standard practice to place an inferior vena cava filter prior to PTE. PTE is performed during circulatory arrest, under deep hypothermia, via a median sternotomy. Following a proximal pulmonary artery incision, all dissection occurs within the pericardium and neither pleural cavity is entered. Loose thrombus is removed and a dissection plane is established within the media of the artery [6]. The dissection plane is then followed circumferentially from the main pulmonary arteries to the subsegmental branches. The procedure is usually performed within 15–20 min of circulatory arrest (Fig. 4.1).

Reperfusion is followed by a second period of circulatory arrest to allow completion of thromboendarterectomy in the contralateral lung [7]. Additional cardiac procedures can be performed after arteriotomy closure, during rewarming, if necessary (e.g. coronary bypass grafting, foramen ovale closure, mitral valve repair). The use of selective antegrade cerebral perfusion for pulmonary endarterectomy appears to be technically feasible in preliminary trials and is a potential alternative to complete circulatory arrest [8].

The Jamieson intra-operative classification of CTEPH defines patients according to the surgical specimens obtained. There are 4 so called "types". In type 1 fresh thrombus is present in the main-lobar pulmonary arteries; in type 2 there is intimal thickening and fibrosis proximal to the segmental arteries; in type 3 there is disease within distal segmental arteries only; in type 4 there is distal arteriolar vasculopathy without visible thromboembolic disease (i.e. misdiagnosed IPAH) [9].

There have been no randomised controlled trials to support the insertion of inferior vena cava filters at the time of PTE and the level of evidence for recommending their use is low [2].

Outcomes of PTE

PTE can be performed with low perioperative mortality, with significant improvements in functional capability, hemodynamics and survival. In-hospital mortality is now <5 % in experienced centres [2]. In the majority of cases post-PTE, there is an immediate and sustained fall in pulmonary artery pressure and pulmonary vascular resistance, with a parallel increase in pulmonary blood flow and cardiac output. There is rapid normalisation of right ventricular geometry and tricuspid valve function, such that tricuspid annuloplasty is not routinely indicated.

The most significant complications of the procedure are reperfusion pulmonary oedema and persistent pulmonary arterial hypertension. Reperfusion oedema most often develops within 72 h of surgery, and corresponds to anatomic locations distal to where PTE is performed [10]. Mechanical ventilation, inhaled nitric oxide (NO) and intravenous iloprost are advocated to improve the oedema. Up to one third of patients undergoing PTE require >2 days ventilatory support because of reperfusion injury, and this complication is responsible for approximately half the mortality associated with the procedure [11].

Persistent pulmonary hypertension, suggestive of inadequate endarterectomy or underlying small vessel/microvascular disease, is a key determinant of short and long term outcomes. Patients with an elevated post-operative PVR have difficulties weaning from cardiopulmonary bypass, early postoperative hemodynamic instability and early postoperative death, particularly in the context of right ventricular dysfunction [2]. Mortality amongst patients with a postoperative PVR exceeding 500 dyn/s/cm^{-5} (6.25 WU) is around 30 times greater than for those with a postoperative PVR of less than 500 dyn/s/cm^{-5}. Although postoperative PVR is the greater predictor of mortality, preoperative PVR in excess of 1,000 dyn/s/cm^{-5} (12.5 WU) has also been associated with poor outcomes [12].

Patients with distal thromboembolic disease (intraoperative classification type 3–4) have higher perioperative mortality, require longer inotropic support, and have longer hospital stays than patients with type 1 or 2 thromboembolic disease [13].

Overall mortality for PTE is reducing with increasing experience of the procedure and is currently less than 5 % [12], with long-term survival exceeding medical therapy or transplantation and persistent improvements in functional status. Four years after PTE around three quarters of patients are in NYHA class I [14].

Surgical Alternatives to PTE

Small scale observational studies in specialist centres have highlighted a potential role for percutaneous pulmonary balloon angioplasty in the management of patients with CTEPH deemed unsuitable for PTE [15, 16]. The technique, which was initially dismissed in the 1980s, has been demonstrated to reduce mean pulmonary artery pressure and effect improved functional capacity. Reperfusion injury is a recognised complication of the procedure and there have been incidences of wiring perforation of the pulmonary vasculature. Systemic and cerebral embolisation are additional hazards. Transplantation remains the definitive surgical alternative for patients with CTEPH not suitable for PTE.

In the acute setting of submassive/massive pulmonary embolism, there is a role for emergency surgical thrombectomy, in preference to thromboendarterectomy. When surgical intervention is contraindicated, percutaneous interventions for removing pulmonary emboli and decreasing thrombus burden include aspiration thrombectomy, thrombus fragmentation, and rheolytic thrombectomy [17].

Atrial Septostomy

Atrial septostomy was originally conceived as a treatment for transposition of the great arteries in neonates [18, 19]. A role for septostomy in the management of pulmonary hypertension was considered when patients with Eisenmenger's syndrome and idiopathic pulmonary arterial hypertension (IPAH) with a patent foramen ovale were noted to have a survival advantage over those without a patent foramen ovale [20]. The first reported use of atrial septostomy in the palliative treatment of refractory primary pulmonary hypertension was in 1983 [21].

Atrial septostomy involves the formation of an intra-atrial right-to-left shunt, diverting blood flow to bypass the pulmonary vasculature, decompressing the right heart, increasing left ventricular preload and augmenting systemic blood flow (particularly during exercise). The resulting increase in cardiac output enhances tissue perfusion, albeit with a reduced systemic arterial oxygen saturation.

Severe IPAH is the most common indication for atrial septostomy. The procedure has also been used for patients with pulmonary arterial hypertension associated with surgically corrected congenital heart disease, peripheral CTEPH and connective tissue disease.

Patient Selection

Atrial septostomy is recommended only for patients with severe pulmonary arterial hypertension and intractable right heart failure resistant to maximal medical therapy (including inotropic support) [22]. Evidence suggests a benefit in patients in WHO functional class IV with refractory right heart failure or severe syncopal symptoms.

For optimum benefit, the procedure should be performed before there is advanced end-organ dysfunction and haemodynamic compromise. Contraindications to the procedure are the requirement for cardio-respiratory support, mean right atrial pressure >20 mmHg, pulmonary vascular resistance index >55 WU/m² (where PVRI is defined as the pressure drop across the pulmonary circulation divided by cardiac index), resting oxygen saturation <90 % on room air, and left ventricular end diastolic pressure >18 mmHg [23]. Patient selection therefore requires experience and judgment. If clinically indicated, patients may undergo serial septostomy procedures.

Surgical Technique

Atrial septostomy is performed by surgical incision (the blade technique), graded balloon dilation or a combination of the two. The balloon dilatation technique is preferred as it offers comparable improvements in symptoms and haemodynamics but a lesser procedural risk than the blade technique.

In the balloon dilatation approach, a Swan-Ganz catheter is placed via the right internal jugular vein for haemodynamic monitoring (right atrial pressure, mean pulmonary artery pressure and cardiac index using the thermodilution method). A sheath is passed into the left atrium by needle puncture. Thereafter, a balloon catheter is passed across the septum

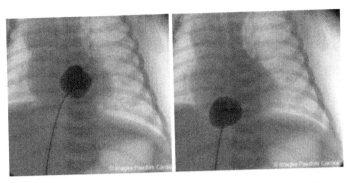

FIGURE 4.2 Balloon atrial septostomy under fluoroscopic guidance (paediatric image) [25]

through the sheath on a guide wire and the sheath withdrawn to the right atrium. The balloon is inflated at low pressures under fluoroscopic guidance. The procedure is repeated with increasing balloon sizes until a septal defect is created that results in a 10 % fall in arterial oxygen saturation [24]. Oxygen delivery is optimised by the transfusion of packed red blood cells or darbepoetin administered pre and post-procedure (Fig. 4.2).

In the blade-balloon approach, balloon dilatation is preceded by the use of a surgical blade, withdrawn across the intra-atrial septum. A total of 3–6 incisions are made at orthagonal angles to achieve a 5–10 % fall in arterial oxygen saturation [26].

The use of intra-cardiac echocardiography to guide the location and extent of septostomy formation has been reported [27]. Recently, a novel septostomy device has been trialled, comprising an atrial septal defect closure device, customised with four 5 mm diameter holes in the central region, but this is not yet in routine use [28].

Outcomes of Atrial Septostomy

There is concern regarding high procedural mortality for septostomy, which is estimated at 16 % but has been reported from 5 to 50 % [29]. Mortality is higher for the blade balloon technique, which carries a greater risk of septal laceration and fatal hypoxaemia. Septostomy is largely restricted to critically ill patients with severe pulmonary hypertension and right ventricular impairment, therefore patient selection contributes to the high mortality. A mean right atrial pressure >20 mmHg, PVR index >55 WU/m^2, and an estimated 1-year survival less than 40 % are significant predictors of procedure-related death [29]. Septostomy is primarily a palliative or bridging procedure and reported success rates for bridging patients to transplantation range from 30 to 40 % [30]. Improved cardiac output appears to be the principal hemo-dynamic benefit. There is an associated symptomatic and functional improvement measured by NYHA class and 6 min walk test [31, 32]. Worldwide experience has demonstrated a median survival of 19.5 months (range, 2–96 months), and late deaths primarily result from progression of underlying pulmonary vascular disease [29].

Surgical Alternatives to Atrial Septostomy

An innovative alternative to septostomy is the Potts shunt procedure, in which needle perforation of the descending aorta is performed at the site of apposition to the left pulmonary artery to create a tract for deployment of a stent between these vessels [33, 34]. The stent acts as a shunt between the pulmonary and systemic circulation, avoiding an intra-cardiac shunt. At present this procedure is limited to the research setting.

Transplantation

The first heart-lung transplant was performed in 1981, for a female patient with IPAH. With the evolution of single and bilateral lung transplant procedures, transplantation is now considered the final definitive treatment for carefully selected patients with advanced pulmonary hypertension. The most common indication is IPAH; less common indications are scleroderma, histiocytosis, and sarcoidosis. Improved disease-specific medical management has reduced the number of patients referred for transplantation; however, around 25 % of patients with IPAH fail to respond to medical therapy.

There is a lack of consensus on the optimal transplantation procedure for patients with pulmonary hypertension. Single lung, bilateral lung and combined heart-lung transplantation have all been performed historically. Single-lung transplantation has been widely discontinued for IPAH due to poor outcomes and International Society for Heart and Lung Transplantation Registry data indicates the majority of pulmonary hypertension patients worldwide receive bilateral lungs. At present, around 5 % of bilateral lung transplants, 3 % of all lung transplants and 28 % of all heart-lung transplants performed worldwide in adults are for IPAH [35].

Patient Selection

Transplantation should be considered and/or discussed with all patients at the time of diagnosis of pulmonary arterial hypertension. Early referral minimises the transplantation of patients with established significant comorbidity. The timing of referral is a recognised challenge given the poor prognosis of patients with disease refractory to medical management and the limited availability of organs.

The International Society for Heart and Lung Transplantation (ISHLT) has published guidelines for the referral and listing of potential transplant candidates. Referral is recommended for patients in NYHA functional class III or IV (irrespective of on-going therapy), or those with rapidly progressive disease. Listing is recommend for patients with persistent functional class III or IV on maximal medical therapy, failure to respond to intravenous epoprostenol (or equivalent), 6 min walk distance <350 m or declining, cardiac index <2 L/min/m^2 and right atrial pressure >15 mmHg.

The majority of patients are listed for bilateral lung transplant. Heart-lung transplantation is reserved for patients with intractable right heart failure, especially those who are dependent on inotropic support. Patients with pulmonary hypertension secondary to congenital heart disease (particularly those with Eisenmenger's) are also more likely to be considered for the combined procedure, although isolated lung transplant may be performed concurrently with cardiac repair. Rarely, the combined procedure is offered to patients with pulmonary hypertension and coexistent advanced left heart disease [36].

Surgical Technique

Anaesthesia in the intended transplant recipient is generally postponed until the donor lungs have been inspected and approved by the retrieval team. The recipient is intubated with a double lumen tube to allow single-lung ventilation. In severe pulmonary hypertension, single-lung ventilation is not attempted. Trans-oesophageal echocardiography is used to monitor right ventricular function and cardiac filling.

Bilateral lung transplantation is typically performed via a transverse thoracosternotomy (clamshell incision). Median sternotomy and bilateral anterolateral thoracotomies with sternal sparing are also used. Bilateral lungs are implanted separately and sequentially. The first lung to be transplanted is generally the one with the least perfusion on V/Q scanning [37].

Cardiopulmonary bypass is often commenced electively in patients with pulmonary arterial hypertension or when concomitant coronary artery bypass graft or cardiac repair is planned. If cardiopulmonary bypass is required for hemodynamic or ventilatory support, the heart remains warm and beating. If cardiac repair is necessary, the heart is arrested and cooled.

Perioperative Considerations

Lung transplantation is associated with an immediate improvement in pulmonary artery pressure with rapid normalisation of right ventricular size and septal geometry [38].

Despite the reduction in right ventricular afterload, right ventricular systolic function and left diastolic function do not improve immediately and haemodynamic instability is common in the early postoperative period. As such, patients with pulmonary arterial hypertension often require temporary inotropic, vasopressor, and inhaled nitric oxide support. Ventricular assist devices are increasingly used to support the right ventricle as it recovers.

In patients without pulmonary hypertension, ventilatory weaning usually occurs over the first few hours to days. In patients with pulmonary hypertension, haemodynamics and oxygenation are more labile, especially following single lung transplantation. A more cautious weaning approach is adopted with the continuation of neuromuscular paralysis, sedation, and ventilatory support for 24–48 h postoperatively. Thereafter, paralysis and sedation are gradually reversed and weaning follows.

Within the first 72 h post-transplant, primary graft dysfunction is a significant concern in patients with pulmonary arterial hypertension, and is associated with increased risk of death [39]. Risk factors for primary graft dysfunction include intraoperative hemorrhage or cardiovascular complications, ischemia-reperfusion lung injury, and the use of cardiopulmonary bypass in the context of severe right ventricular dysfunction. Ischaemia-reperfusion injury is more prevalent following single lung transplantation, when there is a preponderance of blood flow to the allograft lung in response to high pulmonary vascular resistance in the native lung. Any compromise to the allograft (e.g. infection, rejection) can therefore result in severe ventilation-perfusion mismatch [40]. Bilateral lung transplantation results in a lesser degree of ventilation-perfusion mismatch and these patients are easier to care for in the perioperative period.

Outcomes of Transplantation

Survival after lung and heart-lung transplantation for IPAH has historically been lower than for other major diagnostic categories of lung transplant recipients, although higher than

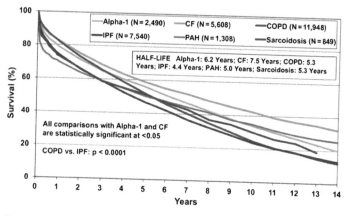

FIGURE 4.3 Kaplan-Meier survival by diagnosis for adult lung transplants performed between January 1990 and June 2010 [35]. (*Alpha-1* α_1-antitrypsin deficiency emphysema, *CF* cystic fibrosis, *COPD* chronic obstructive pulmonary disease, *IPF* idiopathic pulmonary fibrosis, *PAH* pulmonary arterial hypertension)

for idiopathic pulmonary fibrosis. Recent data suggests that although patients with IPAH undergoing transplantation have an increased 3 month mortality, their long term outcomes are comparable with patients with other diagnoses [35, 41].

The ISHLT registry reports 1-, 3-, 5-, and 10-year survival of 66 %, 57 %, 47 %, and 27 %, respectively, in pulmonary arterial hypertension patients undergoing lung transplantation [42]. These compare with baseline survival rates of 79, 64, 53, and 30 % for all lung transplant procedures [35] (Fig. 4.3).

ISHLT registry data demonstrates improved survival amongst all patients receiving bilateral rather than single lung transplant [35] and this is especially the case for IPAH. To date, there have been no direct comparisons of lung transplant versus heart-lung transplant in this population. In patients with Eisenmenger's syndrome secondary to ventricular septal defect, there appears to be a survival benefit with combined heart-lung transplant over bilateral lung transplant with simultaneous closure of the defect.

The incidence of postoperative obliterative bronchiolitis appears to be higher in patients with IPAH and the process onsets sooner than for other conditions necessitating transplantation [43]. Recurrence of IPAH after transplantation has not been reported.

Ventricular Assist Devices

Mechanical circulatory support has a recognised role in the management of left and biventricular failure. In patients awaiting cardiac transplant, left ventricular assist devices (LVADs) have been demonstrated to reduce pulmonary vascular resistance by offloading the left heart [44], nevertheless, acute right heart failure is a not infrequent complication of LVAD implantation [45]. Right ventricular assist devices (RVADs) are effective in RV failure secondary to LV failure and their utility in acute postoperative RV failure is well described [46]. Computational modelling suggests RVAD support can effectively increase cardiac output and decrease right atrial pressure but has the unwanted consequence of increasing pulmonary artery and capillary pressures [47]. Pulsatile mechanical circulatory devices impart significant energy to the circulation, even when the devices are pneumatically driven and set to deliver the lowest possible flow rates. There is an associated risk of damage to the pulmonary microcirculation, with increased pulmonary vascular resistance and pulmonary artery pressure. In patients with pre-existing pulmonary hypertension, RVADs are most commonly used as a bridge to transplantation, although outcomes are anecdotally poor. Alveolar haemorrhage, haemoptysis, and death have been documented [23]. At present, there is insufficient evidence to fully support the use of RVADs in these patients.

Extracorporeal Life Support

Extracorporeal life support (ECLS) is commonly used for adults with acute lung injury and respiratory failure and has been successfully used to treat persistent pulmonary hypertension in neonates [48]. There is a growing body of evidence for the use of ECLS following massive pulmonary embolism and as peri-operative support following PTE for CTEPH (when severe reperfusion oedema is a concern) [49]. ECLS is increasingly used as a bridge to lung transplantation in patients with pulmonary hypertension and in the immediate post-operative period [50, 51].

In patients with pulmonary hypertension and potentially reversible right heart failure, ECLS should be considered when maximal medical management (including targeted PH medication, fluid management, inotropes and optimised ventilation) is insufficient.

ECLS involves the use of a mechanical pump to provide prolonged cardiopulmonary bypass. Blood passes through a heat exchanger and membrane oxygenator where haemoglobin is saturated with oxygen and carbon dioxide is removed. Oxygenation is determined by flow rate, while elimination of carbon dioxide is controlled by adjusting the rate of countercurrent gas flow through the oxygenator [52].

The modality of ECLS selected depends upon specific patient requirements. Veno-venous ECLS (using large bore cannulae sited in the internal jugular or right common femoral vein) is useful for carbon dioxide removal, oxygenation, and right ventricular afterload reduction. Veno-arterial ECLS (from a large vein or the right atrium, returned to the common femoral, common carotid, or right axillary artery) is preferred for right ventricular decompression and after lung transplantation, when the left ventricle may be unable to handle a normalised preload, because it supports the cardiac output and delivers more effective oxygenation [23, 53]. In both forms of ECLS, carbon dioxide removal is superior to oxygenation.

The use of ECLS is currently limited by complications associated with cannulation (pneumothorax, vascular trauma, bleeding, infection, embolisation), systemic anticoagulation, and exsanguination resulting from circuit disruptions. The incidence of clinically relevant complications increases significantly after a period of around 2 weeks. Nevertheless, ECLS remains a potentially lifesaving intervention in patients with right ventricular failure.

The pumpless lung-assist device (LAD) (i.e. Novalung GmbH, Talheim, Germany) has a role in the management of

	VA ECLS	VV ECLS	AV ECLS (Lung Assist Device)
Arterial cannulation	☑	☒	☑
External pump	☑ Lower perfusion rates required	☑ Higher perfusion rates required	☒ Perfusion driven by cardiac output
Gas Exchange	☑ Achieves higher PaO_2	☑ Achieves lower PaO_2	☑ Achieves lower PaO_2
Cardiac Support	☑	☒	☒
Offloading of pulmonary circulation	☑	☒	☑/☒
Example indications	Cardiogenic shock, as a bridge to ventricular assist device or cardiac transplantation	Respiratory failure with preserved cardiac function e.g. ARDS, graft dysfunction post lung transplantation	Severe hypercapnia, respiratory acidosis but moderate hypoxaemia

FIGURE 4.4 Characteristics of VA ECLS, VV ECLS and the lung assist device

patients with predominantly hypercapnic respiratory failure. It operates as a low resistance arterio-venous system, and relies on the patient's cardiac output to drive blood flow. Cannulation of the main pulmonary artery trunk and the left atrium creates a septostomy-like pulmonary vascular shunt, perfused by approximately 20 % of the left ventricular output, contributing to gas exchange and hemodynamic unloading of the right ventricle. An alternative common configuration involves the cannulation of the femoral artery and contralateral femoral vein. The LAD has been successfully used as a bridge to transplantation in selected pulmonary hypertension patients with acute decline attributable to cardiogenic shock [54]. Reports suggest the LAD may be more suitable than ECLS for prolonged use [55] (Fig. 4.4).

Conclusion

- All surgery for pulmonary hypertension should be performed in centres with experience and expertise in these techniques.
- Pulmonary thromboendarterectomy is the only recognised cure for chronic thromboembolic pulmonary hypertension

and should be considered for all patients with the condition.

- Assessment for pulmonary thromboendarterectomy should take precedence over the initiation of medical therapy but inoperable patients should be referred for a trial of medication.
- Atrial septostomy is currently recommended for patients with severe pulmonary arterial hypertension and intractable right heart failure but the procedure may be underutilised.
- The challenge remains to develop methods to ensure an adequate, lasting septostomy.
- Improved disease-specific medical therapy has reduced the number of patients referred for transplantation; however, bilateral lung or heart-lung transplantation remains an important option for selected patients with advanced pulmonary hypertension.
- Referral to a transplant centre is recommended for patients in NYHA functional class III or IV (irrespective of ongoing therapy), or those with rapidly progressive disease.
- At present, there is insufficient evidence to fully support the use of right ventricular assist devices in patients with advanced pulmonary hypertension.
- The development of right ventricular assist devices tailored to the circulatory characteristics of these patients may increase their utility.
- Extracorporeal life support and the lung assist device have a role in the management of life threatening cardiopulmonary failure, following pulmonary thromboendarterectomy and as a bridge to lung and heart lung transplantation.

References

1. Rahnavardi M, Yan TD, Cao C, Vallely MP, Bannon PG, Wilson MK. Pulmonary thromboendarterectomy for chronic thromboembolic pulmonary hypertension: a systematic review. Ann Thorac Cardiovasc Surg. 2011;17(5):435–45. Epub 2011/09/02.
2. Jenkins DP, Madani M, Mayer E, Kerr K, Kim N, Klepetko W, et al. Surgical treatment of chronic thromboembolic pulmonary hypertension. Eur Respir J. 2013;41(3):735–42. Epub 2012/11/13.

3. Kim NH. Assessment of operability in chronic thromboembolic pulmonary hypertension. Proc Am Thorac Soc. 2006;3(7):584–8. Epub 2006/09/12.
4. Pepke-Zaba J, Delcroix M, Lang I, Mayer E, Jansa P, Ambroz D, et al. Chronic thromboembolic pulmonary hypertension (CTEPH): results from an international prospective registry. Circulation. 2011;124(18):1973–81. Epub 2011/10/05.
5. Jenkins D, Mayer E, Screaton N, Madani M. State-of-the-art chronic thromboembolic pulmonary hypertension diagnosis and management. Eur Respir Rev. 2012;21(123):32–9. Epub 2012/03/02.
6. Mayer E, Klepetko W. Techniques and outcomes of pulmonary endarterectomy for chronic thromboembolic pulmonary hypertension. Proc Am Thorac Soc. 2006;3(7):589–93. Epub 2006/09/12.
7. Thistlethwaite PA, Kaneko K, Madani MM, Jamieson SW. Technique and outcomes of pulmonary endarterectomy surgery. Ann Thorac Cardiovasc Surg. 2008;14(5):274–82. Epub 2008/11/08.
8. Thomson B, Tsui SS, Dunning J, Goodwin A, Vuylsteke A, Latimer R, et al. Pulmonary endarterectomy is possible and effective without the use of complete circulatory arrest–the UK experience in over 150 patients. Eur J Cardiothorac Surg. 2008;33(2):157–63. Epub 2007/12/14.
9. Jamieson SW, Kapelanski DP. Pulmonary endarterectomy. Curr Probl Surg. 2000;37(3):165–252. Epub 2000/03/21.
10. Levinson RM, Shure D, Moser KM. Reperfusion pulmonary edema after pulmonary artery thromboendarterectomy. Am Rev Respir Dis. 1986;134(6):1241–5. Epub 1986/12/01.
11. Auger WR, Kerr KM, Kim NH, Ben-Yehuda O, Knowlton KU, Fedullo PF. Chronic thromboembolic pulmonary hypertension. Cardiol Clin. 2004;22(3):453–66. 3. Epub 2004/08/11.
12. Jamieson SW, Kapelanski DP, Sakakibara N, Manecke GR, Thistlethwaite PA, Kerr KM, et al. Pulmonary endarterectomy: experience and lessons learned in 1,500 cases. Ann Thorac Surg. 2003;76(5):1457–62; discussion 62–4. Epub 2003/11/07.
13. Thistlethwaite PA, Mo M, Madani MM, Deutsch R, Blanchard D, Kapelanski DP, et al. Operative classification of thromboembolic disease determines outcome after pulmonary endarterectomy. J Thorac Cardiovasc Surg. 2002;124(6):1203–11. Epub 2002/11/26.
14. Corsico AG, D'Armini AM, Cerveri I, Klersy C, Ansaldo E, Niniano R, et al. Long-term outcome after pulmonary endarterectomy. Am J Respir Crit Care Med. 2008;178(4):419–24. Epub 2008/06/17.

15. Kataoka M, Inami T, Hayashida K, Shimura N, Ishiguro H, Abe T, et al. Percutaneous transluminal pulmonary angioplasty for the treatment of chronic thromboembolic pulmonary hypertension. Circ Cardiovasc Interv. 2012;5(6):756–62. Epub 2012/11/08.

16. Mizoguchi H, Ogawa A, Munemasa M, Mikouchi H, Ito H, Matsubara H. Refined balloon pulmonary angioplasty for inoperable patients with chronic thromboembolic pulmonary hypertension. Circ Cardiovasc Interv. 2012;5(6):748–55. Epub 2012/11/30.

17. Jaff MR, McMurtry MS, Archer SL, Cushman M, Goldenberg N, Goldhaber SZ, et al. Management of massive and submassive pulmonary embolism, iliofemoral deep vein thrombosis, and chronic thromboembolic pulmonary hypertension: a scientific statement from the American Heart Association. Circulation. 2011;123(16):1788–830. Epub 2011/03/23.

18. Blalock A, Hanlon CR. The surgical treatment of complete transposition of the aorta and the pulmonary artery. Surgery, Gynecology & Obstetrics. 1950;90(1):1–15, illust. Epub 1950/01/01.

19. Rashkind WJ, Miller WW. Creation of an atrial septal defect without thoracotomy. A palliative approach to complete transposition of the great arteries. JAMA. 1966;196(11):991–2. Epub 1966/06/13.

20. Rozkovec A, Montanes P, Oakley CM. Factors that influence the outcome of primary pulmonary hypertension. Br Heart J. 1986;55(5):449–58. Epub 1986/05/01.

21. Rich S, Lam W. Atrial septostomy as palliative therapy for refractory primary pulmonary hypertension. Am J Cardiol. 1983;51(9):1560–1. Epub 1983/05/15.

22. Galie N, Hoeper MM, Humbert M, Torbicki A, Vachiery JL, Barbera JA, et al. Guidelines for the diagnosis and treatment of pulmonary hypertension. Eur Respir J. 2009;34(6):1219–63. Epub 2009/09/15.

23. Keogh AM, Mayer E, Benza RL, Corris P, Dartevelle PG, Frost AE, et al. Interventional and surgical modalities of treatment in pulmonary hypertension. J Am Coll Cardiol. 2009;54(1 Suppl):S67–77. Epub 2009/07/09.

24. Reichenberger F, Pepke-Zaba J, McNeil K, Parameshwar J, Shapiro LM. Atrial septostomy in the treatment of severe pulmonary arterial hypertension. Thorax. 2003;58(9):797–800. Epub 2003/08/30.

25. Boehm W, Emmel M, Sreeram N. Balloon atrial septostomy: history and technique. Images Paediatr Cardiol. 2006;8(1):8–14. Epub 2006/01/01.

26. Kerstein D, Levy PS, Hsu DT, Hordof AJ, Gersony WM, Barst RJ. Blade balloon atrial septostomy in patients with severe primary pulmonary hypertension. Circulation. 1995;91(7):2028–35. Epub 1995/04/01.

27. Moscucci M, Dairywala IT, Chetcuti S, Mathew B, Li P, Rubenfire M, et al. Balloon atrial septostomy in end-stage pulmonary hypertension guided by a novel intracardiac echocardiographic transducer. Catheter Cardiovasc Interv. 2001;52(4):530–4. Epub 2001/04/04.

28. O'Loughlin AJ, Keogh A, Muller DW. Insertion of a fenestrated Amplatzer atrial septostomy device for severe pulmonary hypertension. Heart Lung Circ. 2006;15(4):275–7. Epub 2006/07/22.

29. Sandoval J, Rothman A, Pulido T. Atrial septostomy for pulmonary hypertension. Clin Chest Med. 2001;22(3):547–60. Epub 2001/10/10.

30. McLaughlin VV, Archer SL, Badesch DB, Barst RJ, Farber HW, Lindner JR, et al. ACCF/AHA 2009 expert consensus document on pulmonary hypertension: a report of the American College of Cardiology Foundation Task Force on Expert Consensus Documents and the American Heart Association: developed in collaboration with the American College of Chest Physicians, American Thoracic Society, Inc., and the Pulmonary Hypertension Association. Circulation. 2009;119(16):2250–94. Epub 2009/04/01.

31. Sandoval J, Gaspar J, Pulido T, Bautista E, Martinez-Guerra ML, Zeballos M, et al. Graded balloon dilation atrial septostomy in severe primary pulmonary hypertension. A therapeutic alternative for patients nonresponsive to vasodilator treatment. J Am Coll Cardiol. 1998;32(2):297–304. Epub 1998/08/26.

32. Law MA, Grifka RG, Mullins CE, Nihill MR. Atrial septostomy improves survival in select patients with pulmonary hypertension. Am Heart J. 2007;153(5):779–84. Epub 2007/04/25.

33. Esch JJ, Shah PB, Cockrill BA, Farber HW, Landzberg MJ, Mehra MR, et al. Transcatheter Potts shunt creation in patients with severe pulmonary arterial hypertension: initial clinical experience. J Heart Lung Transplant. 2013;32(4):381–7. Epub 2013/02/19.

34. Blanc J, Vouhe P, Bonnet D. Potts shunt in patients with pulmonary hypertension. N Engl J Med. 2004;350(6):623. Epub 2004/02/06.

35. Christie JD, Edwards LB, Kucheryavaya AY, Benden C, Dipchand AI, Dobbels F, et al. The Registry of the International

Society for Heart and Lung Transplantation: 29th adult lung and heart-lung transplant report-2012. J Heart Lung Transplant. 2012;31(10):1073–86. Epub 2012/09/15.

36. Olland A, Falcoz PE, Canuet M, Massard G. Should we perform bilateral-lung or heart–lung transplantation for patients with pulmonary hypertension? Interact Cardiovasc Thorac Surg. 2013;17(1):166–70.

37. Boasquevisque CH, Yildirim E, Waddel TK, Keshavjee S. Surgical techniques: lung transplant and lung volume reduction. Proc Am Thorac Soc. 2009;6(1):66–78. Epub 2009/01/10.

38. Katz WE, Gasior TA, Quinlan JJ, Lazar JM, Firestone L, Griffith BP, et al. Immediate effects of lung transplantation on right ventricular morphology and function in patients with variable degrees of pulmonary hypertension. J Am Coll Cardiol. 1996; 27(2):384–91. Epub 1996/02/01.

39. Whitson BA, Nath DS, Johnson AC, Walker AR, Prekker ME, Radosevich DM, et al. Risk factors for primary graft dysfunction after lung transplantation. J Thorac Cardiovasc Surg. 2006;131(1):73–80. Epub 2006/01/10.

40. Levine SM, Jenkinson SG, Bryan CL, Anzueto A, Zamora CA, Gibbons WJ, et al. Ventilation-perfusion inequalities during graft rejection in patients undergoing single lung transplantation for primary pulmonary hypertension. Chest. 1992;101(2):401–5. Epub 1992/02/01.

41. Toyoda Y, Thacker J, Santos R, Nguyen D, Bhama J, Bermudez C, et al. Long-term outcome of lung and heart-lung transplantation for idiopathic pulmonary arterial hypertension. Ann Thorac Surg. 2008;86(4):1116–22. Epub 2008/09/23.

42. Trulock EP, Edwards LB, Taylor DO, Boucek MM, Keck BM, Hertz MI. Registry of the International Society for Heart and Lung Transplantation: twenty-third official adult lung and heart-lung transplantation report–2006. J Heart Lung Transplant. 2006;25(8):880–92. Epub 2006/08/08.

43. Kshettry VR, Kroshus TJ, Savik K, Hertz MI, Bolman RM. Primary pulmonary hypertension as a risk factor for the development of obliterative bronchiolitis in lung allograft recipients. Chest. 1996;110(3):704–9. Epub 1996/09/01.

44. Zimpfer D, Zrunek P, Roethy W, Czerny M, Schima H, Huber L, et al. Left ventricular assist devices decrease fixed pulmonary hypertension in cardiac transplant candidates. J Thorac Cardiovasc Surg. 2007;133(3):689–95. Epub 2007/02/27.

45. Dang NC, Topkara VK, Mercando M, Kay J, Kruger KH, Aboodi MS, et al. Right heart failure after left ventricular assist device implantation in patients with chronic congestive heart failure. J Heart Lung Transplant. 2006;25(1):1–6. Epub 2006/01/10.

46. Chen JM, Levin HR, Rose EA, Addonizio LJ, Landry DW, Sistino JJ, et al. Experience with right ventricular assist devices for perioperative right-sided circulatory failure. Ann Thorac Surg. 1996;61(1):305–10. discussion 11–3. Epub 1996/01/01.

47. Punnoose L, Burkhoff D, Rich S, Horn EM. Right ventricular assist device in end-stage pulmonary arterial hypertension: insights from a computational model of the cardiovascular system. Prog Cardiovasc Dis. 2012;55(2):234–43. 2. Epub 2012/09/27.

48. Lazar DA, Cass DL, Olutoye OO, Welty SE, Fernandes CJ, Rycus PT, et al. The use of ECMO for persistent pulmonary hypertension of the newborn: a decade of experience. J Surg Res. 2012;177(2):263–7. Epub 2012/08/21.

49. Berman M, Tsui S, Vuylsteke A, Snell A, Colah S, Latimer R, et al. Successful extracorporeal membrane oxygenation support after pulmonary thromboendarterectomy. Ann Thorac Surg. 2008;86(4):1261–7. Epub 2008/09/23.

50. Fuehner T, Kuehn C, Hadem J, Wiesner O, Gottlieb J, Tudorache I, et al. Extracorporeal membrane oxygenation in awake patients as bridge to lung transplantation. Am J Respir Crit Care Med. 2012;185(7):763–8. Epub 2012/01/24.

51. Fischer S, Bohn D, Rycus P, Pierre AF, de Perrot M, Waddell TK, et al. Extracorporeal membrane oxygenation for primary graft dysfunction after lung transplantation: analysis of the Extracorporeal Life Support Organization (ELSO) registry. J Heart Lung Transplant. 2007;26(5):472–7. Epub 2007/04/24.

52. Schmidt M, Tachon G, Devilliers C, Muller G, Hekimian G, Brechot N, et al. Blood oxygenation and decarboxylation determinants during venovenous ECMO for respiratory failure in adults. Intensive Care Med. 2013;39(5):838–46. Epub 2013/01/08.

53. Tudorache I, Sommer W, Kühn C, Wiesner O, Hadem J, Führner T, et al. Lung transplantation for severe pulmonary hypertension--awake extracorporeal membrane oxygenation for postoperative left ventricular remodelling. Transplantation. 2015;99(2):451–8.

54. Strueber M, Hoeper MM, Fischer S, Cypel M, Warnecke G, Gottlieb J, et al. Bridge to thoracic organ transplantation in

‍‍‍‍‍‍‍‍‍‍‍‍‍‍‍‍‍

‍‍‍‍‍‍‍ Patterson

patients with pulmonary arterial hypertension using a pumpless lung assist device. Am J Transplant. 2009;9(4):853–7. Epub 2009/04/07.

55. Bartosik W, Egan JJ, Wood AE. The Novalung interventional lung assist as bridge to lung transplantation for self-ventilating patients – initial experience. Interact Cardiovasc Thorac Surg. 2011;13(2):198–200. Epub 2011/05/06.

Chapter 5
Putting It All Together

Brendan Madden

Awareness among clinicians regarding the clinical manifestations of pulmonary hypertension, the importance of early diagnosis and the development of therapeutic strategies [1–8] has improved considerably. However on-going education is necessary to further improve our knowledge and understanding and to maximise efforts to diagnose the condition early and to define its aetiology.

Pulmonary Hypertension is receiving increasing attention in medical school curriculae and indeed in our unit we have undergraduate medical students performing specialist subject modules in pulmonary hypertension each university term. It is hoped that this will contribute to increasing future awareness among doctors and indeed many of these students have already obtained publications in this area. In addition we have developed an active post-graduate teaching programme for doctors in respiratory medicine, cardiology, intensive care, anaesthesia and cardiothoracic surgery about pulmonary hypertension. To this end local, regional and national study days have been very important. We have also

B. Madden
Division of Cardiac and Vascular Science,
St. George's Hospital, London, UK
e-mail: brendan.madden@stgeorges.nhs.uk

B. Madden (ed.), *Treatment of Pulmonary Hypertension*,
Current Cardiovascular Therapy,
DOI 10.1007/978-3-319-13581-6_5,
© Springer International Publishing Switzerland 2015

171

been pioneering the use of regional study days for nurses to promote increasing awareness of pulmonary hypertension in the community and to promote training of pulmonary hypertension nurses.

Pathways for the diagnosis and investigations of patients with suspected pulmonary hypertension have been established and training of medical staff in techniques such as right heart catheterisation, echocardiographic assessment and radiological imaging have been formalised.

There has been significant advancement in our understanding of the molecular biology of the pathobiology of pulmonary arterial hypertension and this has helped to further our understanding of potential molecular targets for therapeutic Intervention.

It is possible that vascular injury can occur in patients who have a genetic predisposition e.g. bone morphogenetic protein receptor 2 (BMPR2) mutations. If such mutations occur they may lead to a loss of the inhibitory action of BMP on vascular smooth muscle growth. An insult e.g. auto immunity, toxins (not metabolised in patients with liver disease), drugs, and HIV can lead to vascular injury particularly in patients with a genetic predisposition. Endothelial cell dysfunction (e.g. abnormal production of N0, Pg 12, ET-1 etc.) and smooth muscle cell dysfunction (abnormal calcitonin and gastrin releasing peptide metabolism; KV1.5, 5-HTT) can facilitate inflammation (e.g. IL-1, IL-6, chemokines RANTES, fractalkaline and many others) and subsequently vascular remodelling resulting in plexogenic pulmonary arteriopathy.

Although standard initial agents are phosphodiesterase type 5 inhibitors these are frequently supplemented with endothelin receptor antagonists. The indication for these agents alone or in combination with other agents is coming more clearly into focus as treatment guidelines have been developed. Encouraging early experience suggests that macitentan favourably influences prognosis. Furthermore the soluble guanylate cyclase stimulator riociguat will soon become commercially available in the United Kingdom and there is already evidence supporting its use in both pulmonary arterial hypertension and in chronic thrombo-embolic pulmonary hypertension. Subcutaneous treprosti-nil, nebulised nitric oxide and nebulised and IV prostacyclin analogues are routinely used and oral prostacyclin formu-lations are now available. It is becoming clear which patients with other disease processes should and should not be considered for advanced pulmonary vaso-dilator therapy. For example patients with left heart failure may experience an acute deterioration if increasing pulmonary perfusion leads to an acute on chronic elevation of left atrial filling pressure. Additionally there is no proven ben-efit for prescribing this type of therapy for patients with smoking related lung disease when pulmonary hyperten-sion is proportionate to their pulmonary pathology. Furthermore the importance of diagnosis, evaluation and treatment of pulmonary hypertension at pre-operative anaesthetic assessment is now well recognised.

It is also now accepted that patients with pulmonary hypertension should be managed within the confines of a specialist centre. It may be that patients will be seen within the specialist centre exclusively or increasingly, specialist cen-tres are combining with satellite units to offer a joint care service. Such arrangements where protocols are unified have many advantages. Patients can be managed locally in a famil-iar environment by clinicians who are known to them. With clearly defined protocols for diagnosis and work up, appro-priate investigations including right heart catheterisation may be performed in the satellite centre. Under joint care arrangements patients are reviewed at least 3 monthly in joint pulmonary hypertension clinics with representation from clinicians and specialist nurses from both units in attendance.

It is helpful that should a patient from the satellite clinic become acutely unwell they can be admitted locally, where they are known, and treated as appropriate with agreed protocols and discussion with the specialist centre as neces-sary. Often designated pulmonary hypertension centres are stand-alone cardiothoracic units and therefore will not have local support to manage other potential issues which may co-exist in the pulmonary hypertension patient e.g. connective tissue disease, complex haematological abnormalities, rheumatological conditions and hepto-renal disorders. Additionally there may not be an obstetric service for pregnant women who have pulmonary hypertension. For these reasons joint care agreements are usually well received by patients and operate successfully. The experience of the Royal Brompton Hospital and St Georges Hospital has been excellent in this regard over the past 5 years. The development of the role of the pulmonary hypertension specialist nurse has been a significant advancement in the multidisciplinary team management of the patient with Pulmonary Hypertension.

Close communication with surgeons and anaesthetists when patients with Pulmonary Hypertension require surgical intervention is essential. This ensures that the patient is managed in an appropriate environment, that appropriate work-up and treatment strategies are defined and if required a joint discussion regarding the best approach to surgery e.g. open versus laparoscopic approach can take place. Furthermore close communication peri-operatively ensures that should a pulmonary hypertensive crisis develop appropriate information can be given to staff who have previously been made aware of potential complications. Whenever possible, patients with congenital heart disease should be managed in a congenital heart disease centre.

There are a variety of potential surgical options for selected patients who have pulmonary arterial hypertension. Initially experience was with heart and lung transplantation although driven by the well documented shortage of donor organ availability the surgical procedure of choice subsequently became bilateral lung transplantation. Some encouraging experience was reported with single lung transplantation however it was not uncommon for patients to experience often fatal pulmonary oedema peri-operatively which was multi factorial in origin reflecting exposure of the donor organ to brain stem death factors, the influence of organ ischemic time and preservation techniques, discontinuous lymphatic circulation in the recipient, re-perfusion with the recipients blood and the significant disproportion in the recipient between the pulmonary vascular resistance of the native and transplanted lung. With bilateral lung transplantation the pulmonary vascular resistance in both lungs is equal. In addition to the shortage of donor organs, obliterative bronchiolitis post-transplantation remains a major obstacle to be overcome. Pulmonary thrombo-endarterectomy is an option for some patients with chronic thrombo-embolic pulmonary hypertension and is associated with low peri-operative mortality and significant improvement in functional capability, haemodynamics and survival. It should be performed in specialist centres. There may be some role for percutaneous pulmonary balloon angioplasty in patients who are unsuitable for this form of surgery. Atrial septostomoy which was originally developed as a treatment for transposition of the great arteries in neonates can be applied to patients who have severe idiopathic pulmonary arterial hypertension in an attempt to offload the failing right ventricle. It is however a temporary situation and may for some patients be a bridge to transplantation. The precise role for ventricular assist devices and extra corporeal life support modalities in patients with pulmonary hypertension remains to be clarified. Nevertheless it would appear that these treatments have a role should the patient develop an acute reversible condition amenable to therapeutic intervention or require them as a bridge to lung transplantation.

It is hoped that ongoing progress will continue to be made for patients who have pulmonary hypertension and that with increasing awareness, earlier diagnosis will be made. As our understanding of the pathophysiology of the condition improves and our identification of molecular biological targets grows it is logical to expect that newer, more specific drugs will be developed. Futhermore the role of combination therapy will be more clearly defined. Surgery remains an option for a small number of selected patients.

References

1. Bacon JL, Peerbhoy MS, Wong E, Sharma R, Vlahos I, Crerar-Gilbert A, Madden BP. Current diagnostic investigations in pulmonary hypertension. Curr Respir Med Rev. 2013;9(2):79–100.
2. Madden BP. Pulmonary hypertension. In: Yusuf S, Cairns J, Camm J, Fallen E, Gersh B, editors. Evidence -based cardiology. Blackwell Publishing; 2010. p. 1118–31.
3. Madden BP. Pulmonary hypertension and pregnancy. Int J Obstet Anesth. 2009;18:156–64.
4. Ranu H, Smith K, Nimako K, Sheth A, Madden BP. A retrospective review to evaluate the safety of right heart catheterisation via the internal jugular vein in the assessment of pulmonary hypertension. Clin Cardiol. 2010;33(5):303–6.
5. Ranu H, Buyck H, Willis F, Madden BP. Breathlessness and chest pain in a patient with sickle cell disease. BMJ. 2011;343:d3797. (Endgames).
6. Madden BP, Sheth A, Ho T, Kanagasabay R. A potential role for sildenafil in the management of perioperative pulmonary hypertension and right ventricular dysfunction following cardiac surgery. Br J Anaesth. 2004;93(1):155–6.
7. Madden BP, Radley-Smith R, Hodson M, Khaghan A, Yacoub M. Medium term results of heart and lung transplantation. J Heart Lung Transpl. 1992;11:S241–3.
8. Madden B, Hodson M, Tsang V, Radley-Smith R, Khagani A, Yacoub M. Intermediate term results of heart-lung transplantation for cystic fibrosis. Lancet. 1992;339:1583–7.

Index

B. Madden (ed.), *Treatment of Pulmonary Hypertension*,
Current Cardiovascular Therapy,
DOI 10.1007/978-3-319-13581-6,
© Springer International Publishing Switzerland 2015

Printed by Printforce, the Netherlands